1984

Violence in the Medical Care Setting

A Survival Guide

Edited by
James T. Turner

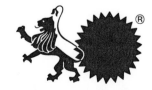

AN ASPEN PUBLICATION®
Aspen Systems Corporation
Rockville, Maryland
Royal Tunbridge Wells
1984

Library of Congress Cataloging in Publication Data
Main entry under title:

Violence in the medical care setting.

Includes bibliographies and index.
1. Hospitals—Security measures. 2. Violence in hospitals.
3. Hospitals—Safety measures. I. Turner, James T. [DNLM: 1. Health
Services—organization & administration. 2. Personnel Management.
3. Violence. W 84.1 V795]
RA969.95.V56   1984   362.1′1′068   84-16840
ISBN: 0-89443-554-X

Publisher: John R. Marozsan
Associate Publisher: Jack W. Knowles, Jr.
Editor-in-Chief: Michael Brown
Executive Managing Editor: Margot G. Raphael
Managing Editor: M. Eileen Higgins
Editorial Services: Ruth McKendry
Printing and Manufacturing: Debbie Collins

Library of Congress Catalog Card Number: 84-16840
ISBN: 0-89443-554-X

Printed in the United States of America

1   2   3   4   5

Table of Contents

Preface

As violence becomes a prevalent form of communication in our culture, health care is experiencing the backwash of this tide. Health care settings, large and small, are under siege. Marked increases in theft, rape, and assault are facts of daily life. A 1982 survey by *Hospital Security and Safety Management*[1] indicates that violent crimes are second only to theft in frequency of occurrence in the hospital setting. A survey by the International Association for Hospital Security reveals that almost all hospitals can expect to experience episodes of violent behavior.[1] Information presented at Congressional hearings concerning federal hospitals for the period fiscal year 1977 to 1980 revealed the following increases in reported incidents:[2]

Robbery	16 percent
Rape	33 percent
Assaults	27 percent
Physical Arrests	16 percent

Often, a wall of silence is erected around such incidents. Fear of negative publicity and increasing staff discomfort contributes to this silence. Denial allows administrators and professionals to believe that these things will not happen in their facilities. The purpose of this book is to encourage open dialogue on violence in health care. Our goal is to open these issues to research and to provide practical information for health care staffs.

Hospitals and related health care facilities are the last open facilities in our culture. Today, even many churches are locked except during services. Yet health care facilities and staffs maintain environments where individuals can move with relative freedom. Visitors frequent facilities with minimal controls. Sick patients under stress enter the private practice office. The basics of personal identification are often ignored; anyone in a white coat can circulate freely.

Data on violence in health care is extremely difficult to obtain. Each of the authors who contributed to this volume faced a formidable task as a result of the limited information available. In some cases, administrators and professional staff members are unwilling to discuss issues formally. In other instances, the lack of a focal reporting point hinders the gathering of information.

Health care facilities—hospitals, outpatient clinics, emergency medical centers, and mental health centers—assume responsibility not only for the treatment of patients, but also for the safety and well-being of patients, visitors, and staff members. The failure to plan for that safety has proven costly in other industries[3]. Worker's compensation issues also arise in relation to the safety of the work place.[4] Unless staff members are specifically hired to work with dangerous patients, the criminally insane, for example, they have grounds to expect relative safety in their health care roles.

This volume asserts that knowledge and training play significant roles in providing maximum safety. Health care providers need to be aware of the types of behaviors within patient groups and the types of settings that contribute to violent behavior. The management of disturbed behavior is a basic part of organizational planning and training. There is no place for senseless recriminations toward staff members when violence occurs. Instead, training and incident analyses need to become a reqular part of the routine so that future incidents of violence are prevented.

Chapter 1 examines the risks inherent in failing to train staffs. The implications of these risks and some suggestions for dealing with these training issues are examined.

Chapter 2 details in a graphic manner the death of a physician—a man who died merely because he was a symbol of the health care system.

Chapters 3 through 9 present overviews of violence in health care settings and among particular patient groups. Methods of preventing and handling such events are examined.

Chapters 10 and 11 concern the spillover into the health care setting of a political problem—hostage taking. Hostage takings in health care settings have increased since 1981. Health care facilities present a unique opportunity for access, hostage taking, and media coverage. Chapter 10 examines some specific health care-related incidents, and Chapter 11 examines issues of hostage survival.

Chapters 12 and 13 are basic primers for nonsecurity health care professionals. Often, health care professionals are in administrative positions which carry responsibility for physical security and program analysis. They may be required to request or approve expenditures for security plans, without really understanding the need for, or the adequacy of, the plans. Chapter 12 presents basic security concepts and their applications. Chapter 13 explores the growing area of personal distress devices.

Chapter 14 examines staff training that does *not* emphasize physical management of the patient. When it becomes necessary for staff members to fall back on choke holds or throws to protect themselves, a basic flaw in the system exists. The risk some systems take in training staff members to rely on physical management without adequate refresher training is not only frightening, but engenders a confrontational atmosphere. With basic training, staff members can develop physical and body language de-escalation techniques that are more than adequate.

Chapter 15 represents another area of fresh ground. To our knowledge, little research has been done on staff victims of violence. In her chapter, Gail Pisarcik Lenehan examines the issues and develops recommended actions for treatment plans.

Violence in the medical care setting takes a heavy toll on fiscal and human resources. Increasing sophistication in health care and attention to technical treatment has led to a loss of the human engineering factor in medical care. Whether it is a physician managing an angry patient, a nurse with an upset family member, a mental health professional with an emotionally disturbed patient, or security personnel with an outsider, the professional's skill in people management determines the outcome in most cases.

This volume provides basic information to practitioners in medical settings so that they can meet the challenge and survive in the face of increasing violence. The alternative is to pull away from our patients, to place more barriers between them and us, and to lose the characteristics of compassion, care, and sensitivity that our patients need so desperately in today's world.

As you journey through the pathways of this volume, fight your own tendency to deny that it could happen to you. As you review the material, apply some of the ideas to your work. The risk is minimal, and the pay-off can be generous. If what you're doing isn't working, don't just do it harder. Try something different.

NOTES

1. R. R. Rusting, "Introduction," in *The Health Security Crisis Handbook*, ed. S. Taitz (Port Washington, New York: Rusting Publications, 1984).

2. House of Representatives, Committee on Veterans' Affairs, Subcommittee on Hospitals and Health Care, *Security Forces at VA Medical Centers* (Washington, D. C.: U. S. Government Printing Office, July 15, 1981).

3. J. Curley, "Suits Charging Lax Security are Increasing," *Wall Street Journal*, October 24, 1983.

4. B. D. Sales, T. D. Overcast, and K. J. Merrikin, "Worker's Compensation Protection for Assaults and Batteries on Mental Health Professionals," in *Assaults Within Psychiatric Facilities,* eds. J. R. Lion and W. H. Reid (New York: Grune & Stratton, 1983).

About the Editor

James T. Turner, Ph.D., holds appointments at the Veterans Administration Medical Center and the Department of Psychiatry at the University of Tennessee Center for the Health Sciences. In addition to maintaining his private practice, he is a consultant to the psychiatric emergency area of the Regional Medical Center. Dr. Turner has presented workshops nationwide on hostage incidents in health care settings. His published articles reflect his broad interest in political applications of psychology. Dr. Turner is a consultant to private industry and federal agencies.

About the Contributors

Lawrence V. Annis, Ph.D., is a clinical psychologist in the Forensic Service of Florida State Hospital. He has worked with convicted sex offenders in Florida and has adjudicated delinquent adolescents in North Carolina.

Christy A. Baker earned master's degrees in anthropology and psychology before becoming an outpatient therapist and the lone psychology resource at a community mental health center in rural North Carolina. She is a doctoral student in the Interdivisional Program in Marriage and Family at Florida State University. Her research focuses on intrafamily violence in different cultures.

Barbara Conwell, M.B.A., earned her degree at the Graduate School of Management at Boston University. She is the director of Unit Management at University Hospital in Boston.

Robert W. Doms, Sr., M.Ed., is a regional manager for Audio Intelligence Devices, Technical Systems Division. A retired lieutenant colonel, Mr. Doms is a lecturer and security consultant to industry and government.

William O. Dyer, Ph.D., is a member of the psychology faculty at Memphis State University. He is the director of the Park Ranger Law Enforcement Training Program for both state and federal park programs. During summer recesses, he combines the academic with the practical as a commissioned federal law enforcement officer. Dr. Dyer provides workshops on security practices for a variety of organizations, including hospitals.

Emily Friedman is a senior field editor of *Hospitals* magazine and a feature writer for American Hospital Publishing, Inc. Ms. Friedman is a sought-after public speaker on health care issues and trends.

Wade Ishimoto is a senior vice president of SAS of Texas, Ltd., based in Austin. Mr. Ishimoto's experience spans two decades of law enforcement, security, and intelligence work. He was one of the Delta Force's primary intelligence officers from its formation through its attempted rescue of

American hostages in Iran. Through SAS of Texas, Mr. Ishimoto recently has been involved in examining for the White House security plans and preparations for the 1984 Olympics.

Radwan Khuri, M.D., is the director of Emergency Psychiatric Services at the Regional Medical Center and an assistant professor in the Department of Psychiatry at the University of Tennessee Center for the Health Sciences. Dr. Khuri is involved in direct service delivery and medical education.

Gail Pisarcik Lenehan, R.N., M.S., C.S., C.E.N., is a psychiatric clinical specialist at Massachusetts General Hospital. She is the editor of *Journal Of Emergency Nursing.* Her research and practice focus on the management of emergency cases and the role of the certified emergency nurse.

Harry A. McClaren, Ph.D., is the chief psychologist at Taylor Hardin Secure Medical Facility, Alabama's primary forensic assessment and treatment center. Previously, Dr. McClaren was a clinical psychologist at Florida State Hospital in the evaluation and treatment of forensic psychiatric patients.

John F. Moran, Ph.D., is the director of Education at Elmhurst Memorial Hospital in Elmhurst, Illinois. Dr. Moran is the editor of *Healthcare Protection Management* and the vice-president of the International Healthcare Safety and Security Foundation. He has presented workshops on aggression management for health care staffs worldwide.

Dan S. Murrell holds both the juris doctor and the master of laws degrees. He is a full professor in the Cecil C. Humphreys School of Law at Memphis State University. Mr. Murrell is a consultant in legal training for law enforcement and has been admitted to the local bar association and courts, and the federal courts, including the U.S. Supreme Court.

William M. Petrie, M.D., is in private practice in Nashville, Tennessee. He is an associate clinical professor at the Vanderbilt Medical Center and a consultant to the National Institute of Mental Health. His research focuses on geriatrics and psychopharmacology.

Dwayne Piercy, Ph.D., is a staff psychologist at the Colmery-O'Neil Medical Center in Topeka, Kansas. For a number of years, Dr. Piercy was the coordinator of alcohol programing and treatment for mixed substance abuse at the Veterans Administration Medical Center, Memphis, Tennessee. He now works in the area of substance abuse prevention and health psychology.

Stephen N. Schilt, M.D., is a board-certified child psychiatrist who has worked in various military settings. He is the chief of the Child Guidance Service at the Madigan Army Medical Center in Tacoma, Washington.

Thomas Strentz, M.S.W., is a special agent for the Federal Bureau of Investigation. He is recognized worldwide as an authority on hostages and the Stockholm Syndrome. Mr. Strentz lectures internationally and has published a number of articles on the Stockholm Syndrome. He is assigned to the Special Operations and Research Section of the FBI Training Academy.

Kenneth Tardiff, M.D., M.P.H., is the associate dean and an associate professor of psychiatry and of public health at Cornell University Medical College. Widely published in the area of violence and psychiatric patients, Dr. Tardiff recently has completed guidelines on the restraint and seclusion of patients for the American Psychiatric Association.

Keith A. Wood, Ph.D., is the chief psychologist for Emergency Psychiatric Services at the Regional Medical Center. He is also an assistant professor in the Department of Psychiatry at the University of Tennessee Center for the Health Sciences.

Don Wright is an inspector and the deputy commander of Field Operations in the Shelby County Sheriff's Department in Tennessee. His law enforcement credentials include graduation from the FBI National Academy. Mr. Wright is involved in the development and implementation of law enforcement training programs for individuals working in institutional settings.

Anthony C. Zold, Ph.D., received his doctorate in child-clinical psychology from the University of Minnesota. He is chief of the Psychology Service at Madigan Army Medical Center, where he established and directs a postdoctoral fellowship in child-clinical psychology.

Chapter 1

Training for Hospital Security: An Alternative to Training Negligence Lawsuits

William O. Dyer, Ph.D., Dan S. Murrell, J.D., LL.M.,
and Don Wright

It is clear that administrators in medical care settings must be prepared to deal with the possibility of violent behavior within their institutions. This preparation involves a whole spectrum of concerns, such as emergency evacuation plans, security procedures, bomb threats, liaisons with law enforcement agencies, electronic security systems, and the selection, training, and deployment of personnel within the institutions. Unfortunately, it is in this last area that many hospital settings fall short in their efforts to deal with violence and inappropriate behavior.

Depending upon the size and location of the medical care setting, provisions for security range from a total reliance on the common sense of professional staff and assistance from local police agencies to sophisticated hospital police units with extensive training and law enforcement authority. The hospital organization may also include specialty wards for psychiatric patients or prisoners, which increase the risks of violence. Some hospital administrators contract with local guard services, hoping that they will be able to provide the necessary protection services in any situations that may arise.

Although there are some notable exceptions, the people placed in these high-risk positions often do not possess the knowledge, skills, and abilities necessary to handle nonroutine situations requiring positive action. This lack of preparation is rooted in several factors: (1) It is commonly assumed that nonroutine incidents are rarely encountered in hospital settings. (2) Administrators often are unaware of what is required to adequately prepare and train their staffs. (3) Training costs time and money. (4) Administrators take an "it can't happen here" attitude toward occurrences of violence and unlawful behavior in their hospital settings. (5) Administrators are reticent to create what they fear will be high security profiles within the walls of their institutions.

1

There are, however, definite risks attendant to a lack of adequate preparation for the eventuality of violence. An obvious risk involves personal injury and the loss of life and property. Certainly, the specter of an occurrence similar to the hostage incident at St. Jude Children's Research Hospital in Memphis in 1982 must create a great deal of anxiety for any hospital administrator. Another issue associated with inadequate preparation involves the legal problems surrounding an area of vicarious liability known as training negligence.

With respect to training for the management of violent behavior, hospital administrators must consider two separate areas. The first involves training for hospital security police, and the second involves training for other hospital staff members, such as physicians, nurses and orderlies, in the management of violent or criminal behavior.

VICARIOUS LIABILITY IN HOSPITAL SECURITY

In the context of this chapter, vicarious liability refers to the legal concept that hospital administrators may be held personally liable for the acts of employees that they supervise, even though they may not have been present when the acts were committed.[1] This type of liability rests on the assumption that the administrators were negligent with respect to some aspect of their personnel responsibilities and that their negligence was the *proximate cause* of injuries inflicted by officers upon citizens. Within the realm of vicarious liability, hospital administrators are at risk in five distinct areas:

1. Negligent appointment: when administrators knew or should have known that individuals they hired were incompetent to carry out their jobs
2. Negligent retention: when administrators knew or should have known that employees were incompetent and should have been dismissed, but were not
3. Negligent assignment: when administrators knew or should have known that employees were assigned to a particular duty or placed in a capacity in which they were incompetent or not prepared to serve
4. Negligent supervision: when administrators knew or should have known that employees required supervision that they did not receive
5. Negligent training: when administrators knew or should have known that employees were in need of certain training for their jobs, but failed to provide it.

Within these five areas, negligence can be divided into two categories:

1. Simple negligence refers to an act or omission that results in a loss.
2. Gross negligence reflects a willful or wanton disregard for any consequences that could reasonably be expected to result from an act or omission.

Furthermore, there are two types of liability that an administrator can incur.

1. Criminal liability is incurred when a person engages in a public wrong within the jurisdiction. The act must both be wrong and carry a penalty. It may be directed against the government, persons, or property. Robbery and murder are examples of such acts.
2. Civil liability results when a person wrongs another—that is, commits a tort. The act may or may not be a violation of some criminal statute, but has a remedy in civil action. The injured party (plaintiff) can attempt to right the wrong through a civil action in court. If the plaintiff demonstrates through a "preponderance of the evidence" that the defendant did in fact wrong him, the plaintiff may obtain relief in the form of a financial award, an injunction, or specific performance. Financial awards may be compensatory and punitive:
    1. Compensatory damages are known as actual damages. They involve money awarded to the plaintiff—actual expenses accrued as a result of the tort—and also may include compensation for pain and suffering, and the loss of a right.
    2. Punitive damages are levied against the defendants in cases where the court wishes to punish them and deter them or others from engaging in similar acts in the future. Unlike actual damages, punitive damages will not be paid by an employee's corporate or municipal entity. Punitive damages come out of the defendants' own pockets.

Since it is civil liability, rather than criminal liability, that typically would be of most concern to hospital administrators, it will be emphasized in our discussion. In doing this, however, we do not wish to devalue the importance of criminal responsibility.

In each of the five areas of vicarious liability mentioned above, case law is rapidly developing that should give all rational hospital administrators reason to reassess their particular situations. In this chapter, we will deal primarily with the last of these areas—training negligence and its potential liability.

What Is Training Negligence?

Consider a hypothetical example in which a hospital security officer with inadequate training uses excessive force to arrest a visitor who he believes has committed a crime. Upon later examination, it appears that the injured visitor's activity was, in fact, not illegal. Or, suppose that an officer failed to take action, the result of which was injury to some innocent party. What are some of the possible outcomes of these incidents? Of course, any criminal charges, state or federal, could be brought against the security officer. An assault and battery might be upheld by the state or federal government as a violation of a citizen's civil rights. The officer may also face civil action in state or federal court as the citizen attempts to recover actual and punitive damages as a result of the officer's action or lack of action, depending on the nature of the injury. In the case of a civil suit, it is also likely that the officer's supervisory chain, including the chief administrator, and the hospital itself, may be named in the suit. The justification for naming all of these other parties is that they were involved in the proximate cause of the incident because they either knew or should have known that the officer lacked the necessary training or background to react appropriately in that particular situation. In other words, they could be guilty of training negligence.

In summary, to perform any job effectively, certain knowledge, skills, and abilities are required. To avoid the significant public relations and legal problems associated with training negligence in institutional security, it is incumbent upon administrators to be aware of the vast array of knowledge, skills, and abilities required for successful performance in the management of violent and criminal behavior and to ensure that the people occupying those positions have been properly selected and trained. It is also wise to ensure that, once trained, those individuals are adequately supervised and that they properly discharge their duties. A review of some recent court actions in the area of training negligence in security and law enforcement should make it quite obvious to any hospital administrator that to overlook the training function is to court serious legal consequences.

OVERVIEW OF CIVIL LIABILITY IN TRAINING NEGLIGENCE

Traditionally, governmental entities and similar institutions and their personnel have been protected from liability under the doctrine of sovereign immunity. In recent years, however, the protective cloak of sovereign immunity progressively has been eroding. This is especially true with reference to the ministerial functions of government—those activities that government engages in to implement its policies and decisions. Common law tradition and public policy recognize the unique nature of the sovereign's activities, such as policing, educating, providing medical services, fire services, transportation, utilities, and the removal of waste. The nature and duty of this responsibility seems to necessitate a degree of immunity from liability because of the nature, hazard, nonprofit character, and unusual care required. On the other hand, any abuse of the office—extreme or gross negligence in carrying out the duties, or simply ignoring the responsibilities of the office—subjects persons who are acting under color of law to liability.[2,3] (Color of law refers to a person's appearing to be or actually being hired by a public entity to enforce the law.) Furthermore, this liability seems to extend from the actor to the responsible supervisor to the legal entity that knew or should have known of the negligent conduct or inaction [4,5] or that failed to correct the situation or prevent a person from being harmed.[6,7] Other public entities have similar responsibilities and duties.

If citizens feel they were wronged by hospital staff members, there are several avenues open to them through which they may pursue civil remedies, depending upon whether the hospitals involved are public or private. One avenue commonly used by people who feel their civil rights have been violated by the action of officers acting under color of law is found in Title 42 of the United States Code (42 USC 1983), Section 1983, hereinafter referred to as 1983. This law, enacted in 1871, provides for civil relief in federal court for people who were deprived of their Constitutionally guaranteed civil rights, privileges, and immunities by officers acting under color of law of a state or territory. There is also a provision for action against a particular individual and against the federal government and its employees. The actual text of the statute reads as follows:

> Every person who, under color of any statute, ordinance, regulation, custom, or usage, of any State or Territory, subjects, or causes to be subjected, any citizen of the United States or other person within the jurisdiction thereof to the deprivation of any rights, privileges, or immunities secured by the Constitution and laws, shall be liable to the party injured in an action at law, suit in equity, or other proper proceeding for redress.

Thus, any hospital security officer operating under color of law is potentially liable under 1983. But what about the supervisors, administrators, and their entities? Are they also liable under 1983?

Common law tradition and public policy entitles officials to a qualified good faith immunity from liability for unconstitutional acts of their employees under 1983. However, since the United States Supreme Court set a new precedent in *Monell*[2] and *Wood*,[3] officials are not immune from such liability if they knew or reasonably should have known that their official actions would result in the violation of someone's Constitutional rights. The very purpose of 1983 is to provide a remedy for police abuse of official position.[8,9]

How are supervisors and administrators held liable under 1983? The Supreme Court holds that an entity can act only through its high-level supervisory officials. Thus, city officials, for example, usually are assumed to set the policies involving hiring, training, and supervising the police force, and, accordingly, may be found to be liable for negligence in structuring or enforcing the policies. A municipality acting through its high-level officials occupies a "supervisory position," and there is a precedent for applying 1983 to supervisors and their entities if a certain degree of negligence on their part also can be demonstrated. Grossly inadequate training would fall into this category. If it is found that a supervisor is guilty of simple negligence in training or supervision, court precedent would dictate that negligence not sufficient to invoke 1983 liability.[10,11] However, if a supervisory official exhibits a "deliberate indifference" to the need for training that results in the deprivation of a plaintiff's Constitutional rights, the entity may be liable under 1983. The court has held that "deliberate indifference is in accord with reckless or grossly negligent conduct on the part of the state officials."[12,13] The entity itself may be considered to have actual or imputed knowledge of the almost inevitable consequences arising from nonexistent or grossly inadequate training and supervising of law enforcement officers.[14,15]

To hold law enforcement administrators liable under 1983 for the unconstitutional acts of one of their officers requires a causal connection to be established between the administrators' grossly negligent actions and the officers' unconstitutional activities. This connection could be made by establishing the administrators' knowledge, acquiescence, support, or encouragement of misconduct, such as excessive force, sexual misconduct, racist conduct, and selective enforcement of the law.[16] Even the mere fact that administrators are aware of constitutional violations may make them liable under 1983.[17] Similarly, administrators could promulgate policies that would make them liable under 1983. Such actions as making inadequate provisions for training, never initiating disciplinary action for the abuse of force, or making statements to the effect that any officers worth their salt would use force every week all would be examples of grossly negligent official policy and would be actionable under 1983.[18]

Defendants in civil law suits have successfully relied on the defense that simple negligence is not a Constitutional violation, while admitting that gross negligence would be actionable.[19] The distinction between simple and gross negligence has already been introduced. There is a clear and significant difference between these two standards; one requires only a showing of unreasonableness, while the other demands evidence of more reckless, shocking, unjustified, and unreasonable action.[20] With respect to the adequacy of training, however, it would appear that gross and simple negligence are merging. There was a time when gross training negligence was virtually synonymous with no training at all, but recent court cases have greatly extended the definition of what constitutes gross negligence. For example, an officer trained in the use of firearms, but not specifically in night firing in a residential area, was held to be inadequately trained and his entity held liable under 1983.[21]

Thus, negative consequences resulting from either the failure of a protective entity to train its police force or the training of that force in a grossly negligent manner is considered to be a violation of a citizen's Constitutional rights.[22] While an entity cannot be held liable for simple negligent training, it may be held liable for grossly negligent training or a total lack of training.[23] Gross negligence or recklessness is, and should be, the subject of 1983 actions, because, as stated previously, the fundamental purpose of 1983 is to provide a remedy for abuse of official position.[24]

It is important to note that 1983 suits brought against law enforcement officers and their entities deal typically, but not exclusively, with the abuse of force in cases involving brutality, false arrest, and firearms. The theory in these cases is often quite simple: any use of force above that which is required and reasonable for carrying out a legitimate law enforcement function, such as an arrest or removal of an uninvited intruder, is considered to be punishment. The Fifth Amendment to the United States Constitution restricts the government to the use of punishment only through due process of law. Due process includes, but is not limited to, the right to counsel, speedy and public jury trial, cross-examination of witnesses, and freedom from cruel and unusual punishment. The Fourteenth Amendment to the United States Constitution guarantees the rights of due process and equal protection under the law, including protection from state action, to every citizen. Therefore, when officers employ excessive force (punishment), they deprive their victims of their Constitutional rights and protections. The purpose of 1983 is to afford victims some relief in federal court, and such cases have become increasingly popular since the 1960s.

The injury a victim receives need not always result in physical or measured harm. The wrong suffered may be intangible or vague. As an example, courts have traditionally compensated parties in Constitutional lawsuits whose voting rights were infringed. Even if a plaintiff in a voting rights case were unable to establish actual or consequential injury as a result of the loss of the vote, punitive damages would be presumed to flow from the wrong itself. Some federal courts have ruled that substantial nonpunitive compensatory damages may be available to persons who are arrested for peaceful demonstrations, denied the opportunity to practice religion within prisons, unlawfully arrested while delivering lectures on the use of contraceptives, or racially segregated.[25]

The thread that runs through all of these cases is a need for pre-employment selection, adequate preservice and inservice training, and effective supervision. Section 1983 has driven the crack in the sovereign immunity armor and has made it easier for more traditional forms of civil action to be successful where injuries occur.

It generally is suggested that the court will react more quickly in allowing recovery of damages when actual or physical injury occurs. Likewise, deliberate action or inaction—such as condoning improper police behavior, providing no training or inadequate training, knowingly using untested or incorrect procedures, providing no supervision or poor supervision, failing to predetermine fitness and ability, or failure to evaluate performance, ability, and conduct—are all likely to bring decisive court action. As examples, consider the following cases:

A motorist, arrested for public drunkenness when in fact he was suffering a massive stroke, was held in the drunk tank, although the officers knew he was not drunk. The citizen brought an action that was allowed to stand for jury determination as to whether or not a violation of his civil rights under 1983 had occurred.[26]

Although a prisoner may have provoked prison guards by his behavior and insults, the guards' response of grabbing and beating him was excessive and suggested official acquiescence at some level. Since the county could be liable for failure to supervise, and because the lack of proper training was so severe as to reach the level of gross negligence or deliberate indifference, the plaintiff was allowed to proceed with a civil action against the county for deprivation of his Constitutional rights.[27]

In another case, the plaintiff recovered damages from the city after her husband, a police officer, shot her and then committed suicide using a revolver that he was required to carry when off duty. It was found that the city failed to use its own newly established psychological test or to initiate other psychological evaluations through which it could have discovered that the officer was mentally ill and should not have been permitted to carry a weapon.[28] The city was held liable because of its failure to consider the problem of identifying officers who are psychologically unfit to carry weapons. It was determined that the police department's screening of employees was inadequate. The court noted that the department did not test incoming officers to determine their psychological fitness to carry weapons and otherwise perform their duties.[29] The department was supposed to use a system to identify problems in duty performance; however, the system was never validated to show that it was appropriate or reliable. In fact, the system was shown to be deficient, both in theory and practice. Additionally, the department ignored all other signs indicating unfitness for duty and for carrying a weapon.[30]

Two additional examples demonstrate the reaction of the courts to deliberate action or inaction by an entity having supervisory responsibility. In a Nebraska case, Yellowbird, an Indian, was beaten, resulting in the death of her unborn child. She was denied medical attention and was threatened.[31] She was able to prove by a preponderance of the evidence that the city and police officers had caused her injury, but only after her attorney was permitted to show that complaints of misconduct, including excessive force, sexual misconduct, racist conduct, and selective enforcement among the city's police had been made by other citizens in the past. In a Rhode Island case, the court allowed a citizen to correct erroneous pleadings and continue proceedings to recover from a situation in which he was physically and verbally abused by five unknown police officers.[32] This was allowed by the court even though the particular officers were not identified.

While it may seem to be a difficult task to assess damages in many of these cases, the courts appear to be quite liberal and willing to provide awards, both compensatory and punitive. Where compensatory damages are considered, the damages may be assessed on the physical harm suffered, including, but not limited to, ill health, physical pain, and discomfort. Also included are considerations of the extent and duration of injuries, and emotional and mental harm suffered, including fear, humiliation, and mental anguish. Additionally, any violation of substantive constitutional rights and due process of law may be considered. Damage awards must take into account the intended intrinsic dimensions of each constitutional right.[33]

Today, courts simply are more responsive to an injured plaintiff when gross negligence occurs. Accordingly, on a finding for the plaintiff, they will quickly assess compensatory damages, even in cases where the damage is intangible. Perhaps this trend should serve as a message to those who are not in good faith conformance.

It is incumbent upon hospital administrators with authority over security forces to ensure that those forces are carefully selected and adequately trained for their roles as agents of authority. Preemployment testing and evaluation, postemployment training and evaluation, and adequate supervision corresponding to carefully drafted guidelines and policies are the new protective shields. Failure to take these minimal precautions in the highly explosive medical care environment leaves the employee, the negligent supervisor, and the entity facing liability unnecessarily.

Nonsecurity Hospital Staff

We have addressed the importance of adequate training for security and police personnel within the medical care setting; but what about the responsibilities of other hospital staff members when they are faced with violent or criminal behavior? Recently, some concern has emerged over whether hospital staff members, such as physicians, nurses, and orderlies, also should receive training in the management of disruptive, assaultive, and violent behavior. To accompany this concern, there is a growing number of consulting firms ready to provide such training.

There are two relevant issues associated with this type of training:

1. Should these employees be provided self-defense training to protect them from others in the hospital or on its grounds?
2. Should these employees be trained in the management of violent and criminal behavior so they can help to control and prevent such behavior? In other words, to avoid possible liability, should hospital administrators ensure that their employees are trained in nonlethal techniques for releasing themselves from the physical control of assailants and physically controlling the assailants until help arrives?

With respect to the first question, it may be a nice gesture to provide self-defense training to nonpolice hospital staff, but a hospital should not be held liable for not providing it. If staff members are assaulted on hospital grounds, the potential liability would probably be based upon negligent security, not upon the victims' lack of training in martial arts.

The answer to the second question is a little more complicated. If the hospital administration writes into all job descriptions a responsibility for the management of violent behavior, that means each staff member essentially has been delegated a security function. To adequately prepare employees for such a role and to reduce the potential liability that such a responsibility incurs would probably require much more training than any workshop would be likely to provide. If a hospital has a potential problem with the physical control of violent and criminal behavior, it had better rely on a well-trained security unit to manage such behavior. It is important to keep in mind that not all violent behavior in medical care settings comes from unruly psychiatric patients.

Training Hospital Security Personnel

Once hospital administrators understand the importance of providing adequate training for their security personnel, their next step is to find out what skills and abilities security personnel should possess in order to do their jobs effectively. This information is best obtained through a training needs analysis, which is a systematic study of the roles, functions, and tasks comprising the job of a security officer. What tasks are security officers called on to do? What should they be expected to do in unique situations? What are the criteria for successful completion of these tasks? What skills are required in order to complete these tasks? Which of these skills must the officers possess when they are hired, and which can be developed through training? The answers to these questions will depend in part upon the particular medical facility; however, there is a common body of knowledge and skills that all of those who enforce laws must acquire in order to carry out their jobs in a legal and proper manner and to minimize the possibility of training negligence suits.

Constitutional Law

All law enforcement officers acting under color of law must be conversant with Constitutional law pertaining to civil rights and due process, especially as articulated in the Fourth, Fifth, Sixth, and Fourteenth Amendments to the United States Constitution. The already complex relationship between civil rights and law enforcement is further complicated by the fact that security personnel have different rights and responsibilities depending on whether they are commissioned by a public entity and, therefore, are operating under color of law, or are hired by private security companies and are operating within their limited citizen police powers. This distinction often is not clearly understood, but it is of tremendous importance, especially in relation to liability. Do citizen police have the authority to stop, frisk, or detain an individual? May they legally use deadly force to stop a fleeing felon? When they hold individuals until the police arrive, have they actually arrested them? Are they subject to federal criminal penalties under Title 18 of the Unites States Code, Section 242 if they deprive individuals of their civil rights? May they be sued civilly in federal court under 1983 for deprivation of civil rights? May they make an arrest based upon probable cause? If they are commissioned as special officers by a city or a county, does it have any Constitutional effect on their status as citizen police? These questions are not easy to answer, yet they represent issues that could become critical when an enforcement action is taken.

Substantive Law, Regulations, and Policies

Regardless of the status of officers' commissions, they must have a good working knowledge of substantive law and be able to answer the following questions: What constitutes arrest power? What are the elements of an arrest? When may someone be arrested, detained, frisked, or searched? What constitutes "reasonable force"? When and how may defensive equipment be used? How is evidence legally preserved? In order to be prepared for their jobs, all security officers must be familiar with these issues and be able to apply them appropriately in law enforcement encounters. Although this prescription by no means will eliminate the possibility of adverse legal ramifications, it will minimize the likelihood of a successful training negligence suit.

IMPLEMENTING A TRAINING NEEDS ASSESSMENT

In addition to being aware of the standard requisites for all those engaged in law enforcement and security activities, hospital administrators must be cognizant of the particular requirements for officers in their institutions before they can implement successful training programs. Training activities often are dominated by a fascination with new instructional technologies, packaged programs, movies, videotapes, computers, and other gadgets that bring "solutions" to training without providing an understanding of the actual problems that the training should solve. Although training should be relevant to the actual jobs to be done, this fundamental concept is often overlooked in the rush to be faddish and to dispense with training in the quickest and most expedient way.

In the training arena, before administrators say, "We have the solutions," they should ask, "What is the problem?" A thorough training needs assessment will answer this question. What are the job skills necessary for a hospital security officer and how can they be obtained most efficiently? These are the questions administrators must be able to answer if they are to minimize the likelihood of adverse legal action or public reaction.

A training needs assessment is a phasic procedure that is based upon a thorough job analysis. The job analysis answers the question, "What do security officers do, or what could they be asked to do?" This information, which Goldstein, Macey, and Prien (1981) call the "content domain" of a job, is obtained by systematically interviewing job content experts, usually the job incumbents themselves or their supervisors. What eventually results is a list of task statements that, taken together, represent the complete scope of the job of hospital security officer.

In addition to the job content information, the job content experts also provide information on the "element domain" of the job—that is, what knowledge, skills, abilities, or personal characteristics (KSAPs) are necessary for the successful completion of each of the tasks comprising the job? Goldstein et al. (1981) define these KSAPs as follows:

1. *Knowledge*: an understanding of facts and principles related to a particular subject area
2. *Skill*: the capacity to perform acts with ease and precision
3. *Ability*: the power to perform a function, physical or mental
4. *Personal Characteristics*: other characteristics, including personality and interest factors

Goldstein et al. provide some guidelines for writing the task statements and the associated element (KSAP) statements:

Task statements should:

1. be written in a clear, direct, and unambiguous style;
2. describe what the officers do, how they do it, and why they do it;
3. be complete, but not so detailed as to become cumbersome; and
4. be given a final analysis by the training analyst to make sure they are clear, accurate, and cover completely the content of the job.

Element (KSAP) statements:

1. should be reasonably balanced between generality and specificity, containing enough information to lead to specific training content;
2. should not be a mere restatement of the task statement; and
3. should not be too trivial.

Some examples of task and element statements are given below:

Task	*Element*
1. Enforce parking regulations in parking lot	Knowledge of parking citation procedures and guidelines for towing illegally parked vehicles
2. Check intrusion alarm control system	Knowledge of alarm system, alarm placements, and procedures for checking and resetting

Task	*Element*
3. Handle disorderly conduct in emergency room waiting area and elsewhere in hospital	Ability to talk to people who are in emotional states and calm them down; knowledge of restraint and arrest procedures; skill with self-defense techniques; knowledge of substantive law regarding disorderly behavior; knowledge of laws and guidelines regarding the use of force
4. Communicate with the dispatcher by radio	Knowledge of radio procedures and codes; skill in use of walkie-talkies and patrol vehicle radios; ability to speak distinctly
5. Testify in court regarding arrests made and citations issued	Knowledge of courtroom procedure and etiquette; ability to prepare cases, speak clearly, remain calm under cross-examination and project appropriate courtroom demeanor

After the list of tasks and their associated KSAPs have been generated, the next step is to have a group of job content experts rate each of the tasks for (1) importance to the overall job; (2) frequency of occurrence on the job; and (3) difficulty of the task (Goldstein, Macey, and Prien, 1981). These ratings are then collated, and the results are used to help identify those areas of training that should be given more emphasis.

With thorough job analyses at their disposal, the training analysts are able to design recruiting or inservice programs to supply the KSAPs required for the job of hospital security officer. This design procedure begins with the following questions:

1. What KSAPs are necessary for the job?
2. Which of those KSAPs should incumbents possess when they initially are employed?
3. Which can be developed in preservice training?
4. Which can be developed in inservice training?
5. Which can be developed in on-the-job training?

Once the analyst has identified the KSAPs to be developed in training programs, the next step is to design a training curriculum that will:

1. instruct officers in the most efficient procedures through effective teaching techniques and methodologies;
2. emphasize the acquisition of those KSAPs which are (a) most important to the job, (b) used most often in the job, (c) most difficult to acquire, and (d) least likely to be safely and efficiently acquired through on-the-job experience;
3. evaluate the degree to which the trainees have developed and can manifest the KSAPs required for their jobs; and
4. provide for a system of evaluating the training program itself that will serve as a foundation for making changes that may be necessary to improve its effectiveness.

THE MEDICAL SETTING STAFF MEMBERS AS PERFORMING ARTISTS

In this chapter, the myriad training techniques, approaches, audio-visual developments, and gimmicks available to augment training programs will not be addressed. It is important, however, to mention one innovation that should be an indispensible element in all training—role play (Dwyer and Kennedy, 1975; Dwyer & Price, 1983). Interest in role play stems from the belief that reducing violence is fundamentally people management. Especially in hospital settings where the emphasis is likely to be on low-key control, health care professionals and security personnel are asked to walk a fine line between minimal use of formal police powers and maximum effectiveness in dealing with those who engage in inappropriate behaviors. Unlike police officers, state troopers, or sheriff's deputies, hospital personnel do not work for law enforcement agencies. Their success is not measured in terms of the number of arrests they make, citations they write, or court cases they win. Rather, these persons are in the compliance business; they must make minimal use of arrest powers (if they have them), and rely instead upon their informal powers of persuasion and interpersonal abilities.

This skill is actually a performing art. Like actors, staff members play to an audience, and their task is to motivate the audience to behave in certain ways. Like the actor's performance, the staff members' performances are evaluated by the audience—not by the amount of applause, but by the degree of compliance.

A problem with traditional hospital police training is that it emphasizes only the formal power aspects of the job—arrests, handcuffs, nightsticks, and guns. With the exception of a few hours of human relations training, very little effort is expended to help officers develop the interpersonal abilities that are so crucial to their jobs. Since these interpersonal people-management skills amount to a performing art, experience indicates that they should be learned in the same way that any performing art is learned—by performing. Role play training involves the presentation of a series of scenarios in front of the class; in each scenario one of the trainees plays the role of the staff member, and the instructors portray hospital patients or visitors who present some behavioral or law enforcement problem. The trainee's task is to deal with the situation as effectively as possible; immediately afterward, the performance is critiqued by the instructors and the group.

In role play training, the skill of the instructors is critical. Not only must they know how to model the correct law enforcement and people-management behaviors, but they must also be good group leaders, providing realistic situations and getting the trainees emotionally involved. Too often what passes for role play in some law enforcement training programs involves a trainee entering a room and getting "shot" by the instructor, or an "assailant" running into the classroom, "shooting" the instructor, and running out; then the trainees describe the perpetrator. Training experience with hospital police suggests that effective role play means getting the trainee involved in interacting with individuals, calming them and motivating them to comply with some law, rule, or order. Of course, formal power aspects should also be practiced in role play scenarios, but they must be integrated into the larger set of interpersonal skills so vital to successful security and law enforcement functioning.

As mentioned previously, personnel in medical settings are in the compliance and persuasion business; too much reliance on formal power surely will get them and their employers into trouble. Thus, their informal skills of talking, persuading, and motivating must be finely tuned, and that can happen only through extensive role play training. Any alternative eventually is likely to result in a day in court.

SUMMARY

For administrators of medical settings, the development of viable security training programs is obviously part of their overall responsibility for the effective management of violent behavior. Personnel also must be adequately recruited, psychologically screened, selected, and professionally supervised. Even then, some problems are bound to arise. Thus, the administrator's task is not to try to eliminate difficulties, but rather to keep them to a minimum. The role that violent-behavior management plays in medical settings will continue to grow; in many urban areas it has already become vital to hospital functioning. With this growth comes the absolute necessity for a proper training foundation for personnel. In this chapter, an attempt has been made to point out some of the undesirable consequences of ignoring the function of training and to outline a structure for developing and implementing adequate training programs. Like so many other areas of administration, the training function has become increasingly important and has developed into a separate discipline in itself. In the arena of hospital security, it is the wise administrator who pays attention to the role that training has to play and incorporates well-developed security training programs into an overall personnel system.

BIBLIOGRAPHY

Dwyer, W. O. and Kennedy, R. (1975). Role Play: An Effective Approach Toward Recruit Traffic-Stop Training, *Tennessee Law Enforcement Journal* 19: 21-25.

Dwyer, W. O. and Price, J. P. (1983). Recreation Area Law Enforcement as a Performing Art: Some Implications for Park Administrators, *Parks and Recreation Resources* 2: 28-29.

Goldstein, I. L., Macey, W. H. and Prien, E. P. (1981). Needs Assessment Approaches for Training Development, in *Making Organizations Humane and Productive: A Handbook for Practioners*, H. Meltzer, ed., New York: John Wiley.

Macey, W. H. and Prien, E. P. (1982). Needs Assessment: Program and Individual Development, *Personnel Selection and Training Bulletin* 3: 144-152.

CITATIONS

1. *Hill v. Marianelli*, 555 F. Supp. 413 (1982).
2. *Monell v. New York City Department of Social Services*, 436 U.S. 658 (1978).
3. *Wood v. Stricklen*, 420 U.S. 308 (1974).
4. *Monell, Id.*
5. *Popow v. City of Margate*, 476 F. Supp. 1237 (1979).
6. *Black v. Stevens*, 662 F.2d 181 (1981).
7. *Smith v. Heath*, 691 F.2d 220 (1982).
8. *Monroe v. Pape*, 365 U.S. 167, 172 (1960).
9. *Popow, supra* at 1243.
10. *Leite v. City of Providence*, 463 F. Supp. 585, 589 (1978).
11. *Hill, supra.*
12. *Leite, supra* at 590.
13. *Hill, supra.*
14. *Leite*, supra at 591.
15. *Hill, supra.*
16. *Herrera v. Valentine*, 653 F.2d 1220, 1225 (1981).
17. *Black v. Stevens*, 662 F.2d 181, 189 (1981).
18. *Black, Id.* at 191.
19. *Popow, supra* at 1242.
20. *Leite, supra* at 591.

21. *Popow, supra* at 1246.
22. *Herrera, supra* at 1224.
23. *Leite, supra* at 590.
24. *Popow, supra* at 1243.
25. *Herrera, supra* at 1228.
26. *Reeves v. City of Jackson, Miss.*, 608 F.2d 644, 649 (1974).
27. *Owens v. Haas*, 601 F.2d 1242, 1247 (1979).
28. *Bonsignore v. City of New York*, 521 F. Supp. 394, 396 (1981).
29. *Bonsignore, Id.* at 397, 398.
30. *Bonsignore, Id.* at 398.
31. *Herrera, supra* at 1225.
32. *Leite, supra* at 587.
33. *Herrera, supra* at 1227, 1228.

Chapter 2

Who Kills Us? Case Study of a Clinician's Murderer

Lawrence V. Annis, Ph.D., Harry A. McClaren, Ph.D.,
and Christy A. Baker, M.A.

On April 2, 1983, a thirty-three-year-old former mental patient named Raymond Colette Thompson wandered unobserved through a hallway at Lexington County's Devon Hills Mental Health Center. He entered an office and shot to death its occupant, a psychiatrist named Alan Woods. The two had met only once, a month before, for ten minutes.

Regrettably, this is not Mickey Spillane fiction, but an actual occurrence. Such a tragedy raises important questions. What sort of person purposely kills another human being merely because the victim is a mental health worker? How can an event like this be predicted? Can it be prevented? This chapter follows a recommendation by Nancy Allen to psychologically autopsy homicides, looking for causes, motives, and alternatives. It is hoped that careful analysis of this case can help health care workers avoid becoming victims.

This paper examines the events leading to Alan Woods' death in order to discern some answers. The authors, who were professionally acquainted with the murderer, reviewed court testimony, sworn depositions, and other documents of public record concerning Woods' death and his assailant. These reports are integrated here in an effort to form a cohesive picture. In this chapter, names and other nominal identifiers have been changed to protect the parties involved.

Portions of this chapter were presented at the annual convention of the Southeastern Psychological Association in New Orleans, March 29-31, 1984. The assistance of Monte F. Bein in the preparation of this chapter is appreciated.

THE VICTIM

Alan Woods was the elder son of a college English professor and a high school music teacher. He attended Louisiana State University, earned an M.D. at the University of Tennessee, and completed his psychiatric residency in Kentucky. He was on the staff at Washington Hospital Center in the District of Columbia for five years before moving to Devon Hills, where he had been for 18 months before his murder. Married since medical school, he had two daughters and an adopted son. He was an accomplished flutist who had performed with the Lexington Community Symphony, and he had recently begun playing tennis. Alan Woods was thirty-seven years old.

THE MURDERER

Developmental information about Raymond Colette Thompson is sketchy. He was born in 1950, the second of three brothers. The eldest, with whom Thompson's contact was limited even as a child, became an officer in the state highway patrol. His younger brother resided in a group home for psychiatric patients. When Thompson was ten, he had beaten his brother with a fire iron during a fit of anger. The considerable cranial injuries resulted in years of psychiatric hospitalization and an adult who was mentally retarded, sensorially impaired, and institutionalized. Thompson's mother had been ill for some dozen years when she retired from her job as bookkeeper at a large department store in 1975. His father had died in a 1963 car crash.

Thompson was first admitted to nearby Clearbrook Hospital after the 1960 battery on his brother. He was subsequently a mental patient at Clearbrook and on the juvenile psychiatric ward of Lexington's Metropolitan Hospital 12 times, the longest of which lasted four months and the shortest three days. He was variously diagnosed as suffering adjustment reaction of childhood and adolescent major depression, schizotypal personality, and undifferentiated schizophrenia.

Thompson used money from his father's insurance and from his mother to attend college, eventually earning a master's degree in sociology from Lexington College. He later was employed in rather menial jobs for one of his educational attainments, working as a store clerk, stock clerk, and librarian's assistant. Teachers, co-workers, and fellow students considered him a loner, a very private person who kept to himself during the day and was not known to socialize after work or school. His principal interest seemed to be firearms, and he accumulated a large number of high-quality pistols and rifles. In 1976, he severely injured his right arm after reportedly dropping a loaded .45 Colt revolver. Thompson's other consuming avocation was reading. He seemed especially interested in science fiction and the occult.

Thompson's only prior recorded conflict with the law occurred in January 1981. When Thompson offered a check in payment for repairs to his car at a Lexington County garage, the manager advised that the shop accepted cash only. Thompson seemed infuriated, but left the garage after a loud, brief argument. A few minutes later, the manager and customers observed him driving a car from the parking area in front of the shop. They recognized the vehicle as one left for engine tuning by another customer; the keys had been in the ignition. Police were informed immediately.

The bright red Firebird was soon spotted. In the chase that ensued, Thompson reportedly reached speeds in excess of 100 miles per hour. He passed other vehicles by making frequent and erratic lane changes, driving on the road shoulder, and forcing other cars to take violent, evasive action. The chase ended abruptly when the Firebird side-swiped a truck, struck a drainage embankment, and came to rest on its side in three feet of mud. Thompson was still sitting behind the wheel when he was arrested. He was taken to the Lexington County Jail and charged with   reckless driving, eluding arrest by flight, and vehicular grand theft.

Thompson refused to talk to anyone, including his public defender, and rejected consideration of any plea other than not guilty. When psychiatric evaluations were requested, he refused to cooperate with the examiners, stood mute, and was subsequently committed to the secure forensic unit at Central State Hospital as incompetent for trial.

Thompson's contact with reality seemed somewhat tenuous when he was first admitted, despite his good orientation and his denials of hallucinations. His gaze was unusual; he tended to glare directly ahead, his eyeballs unmoving, only sporadically glancing suddenly to one side or the other. He talked in a whisper most of the time, but sometimes raised his voice in unexpectedly loud shouts. Thompson seemed irritable and constantly agitated. He repeatedly threatened peers and staff members, particularly the attending psychiatrist. On one occasion, aides intercepted him as he rushed toward the doctor, fists swinging. Oral medications were generally refused, so he was given injectable Haldol. Thompson was later administered Prolixin intramuscularly. When he refused Cogentin, staff members explained repeatedly and in considerable depth how the drug would prevent extrapyramidal side effects. Nevertheless, he continued to decline anticholinergics, declaring, "I'll tell you when I feel side effects."

This resistance to medications faltered after a month's hospitalization, most of which he'd spent in seclusion, physical restraints, or restricted to the ward's close observation routine. The first sign of approaching competence was when he submitted to biweekly Prolixin injections. After another month, he was described as cooperative and reasonable. He was decidedly eccentric and suffering paranoid ideas, but neither gross hallucinations nor grossly delusional thinking were presented. He seemed eager and able to return to court, and was soon discharged to the Lexington County Jail.

Thompson agreed with his attorney to waive a hearing, and was found not guilty by reason of insanity (NGI). Although most persons found NGI go to Central State Hospital's forensic facility, Thompson, found dangerous to himself or others, was committed to Clearbrook, the nonsecure mental institution of his youth. He also agreed to dispose of his gun collection, and his brother soon sold all the pistols and rifles.

Thompson was described on admission to Clearbrook as hostile and noncompliant. He denied that anything was wrong with stealing a car and claimed he had committed the crime because he was told to by God. Nevertheless, he said he no longer heard voices. Thompson did not appear to be overtly psychotic. Although he avoided group and individual therapy, he was creditably employed in the hospital's patient library. He kept to himself most of the time. After five months, the hospital reported to the court that Thompson was alert, well behaved, and not actively psychotic, and he was ordered discharged. He was diagnosed at the time as a chronic paranoid schizophrenic and antisocial personality. The judge directed that he be placed in a group home in downtown Lexington.

At the group home, Thompson seemed to be constantly reading one book or another. His other principal leisure activity was sleeping. Interactions with his three roommates, other residents, and staff members tended to be superficial and brief, but polite. Despite his previous protests about psychotropics, he rarely missed any of his three daily 10 mg doses of Haldol. He seemed devoted to his paid part-time job in the patient library at Metropolitan Hospital and constantly wore the bright orange windbreaker with the Metro logo.

Thompson paid his first visit to Devon Hills Mental Health Center a few days after arriving at the group home. He was seen by Boyce Bettleman, a psychiatrist, for a medication review, and met his new primary therapist, John Clayton, for the first time. Although Clayton was a psychologist, his principal duties as primary therapist were paper management and quality assurance. Thompson seemed to him to be a case of chronic paranoid schizophrenia in remission, an opinion shared by other mental health workers. Given the patient's history of rejecting psychotherapy, his guardedness during the interview, and the apparently stabilizing effects of the medications, individual or group psychotherapy did not seem indicated. It was, however, recommended that he enroll in the center's Day Hospital, and Thompson subsequently visited there on two or three occasions.

A month after the first medication review, Thompson had a second. This time, the attending psychiatrist was Alan Woods. Woods renewed Thompson's Haldol, and after the ten-minute session wrote that "the patient seems polite and cooperative. Well-organized thinking and no signs of acute distress." Another medication review was scheduled for a month later.

It should be noted that Devon Hills Mental Health Center, then as now, saw about two hundred clients per day in its various program areas. Agitated, disruptive, and combative patients had sometimes been encountered, but none had behaved in an obviously life-threatening manner toward clients or staff. On those rare occasions that help was needed in a treatment room or the lobby, a shout sufficed to bring assistance. Mechanical alarms had been discussed, but were never considered essential. As in most clinics, clients were often found in the halls, traveling between therapists, classes, toilets, lobbies, and the cashier.

Two months after his discharge from Clearbrook, Thompson began his lunch break at Metropolitan Hospital by walking three blocks to KC's Sporting Goods. He told the shopkeeper that he was concerned about crime in his neighborhood and wanted to buy a pistol to protect his home. "I'll just put it in a drawer," he said, "and probably never even use it."

Thompson looked at a number of brand-name guns, and then asked to see cheaper models. He eventually selected a .38-caliber, nickel-plated pistol. The clerk asked him if he knew that the law required a three-day wait between purchasing a handgun and getting possession of it. "Oh, I know all about that," he replied. It was then four days before the murder.

Thompson paid $120 in cash for the weapon, and used his expired and revoked driver's license as proof of his identity. He then returned to work at the hospital. The shopkeeper later testified that Thompson looked no different from the run-of-the-mill customer.

At about that time, Thompson's living area in the group home became decidedly untidy, and his personal appearance began to decline. His baths fell from two or three per day to one or none. His clothing became unkempt, and his long hair went unbrushed. He began to miss his medications. Since other residents sometimes missed their doses, and since Thompson had been such a "regular" at medication dispensing, the event did not seem remarkable at the time.

Thompson also seemed to lose interest in his work at Metro. Tardiness earned him a verbal reprimand from his supervisor. At the group home, he became even less sociable than usual, rarely initiating contacts and abruptly ending conversations by walking away. He was even seen drinking beer at a nearby restaurant, a taboo for residents. The observer, a counseler in another group home, later reported this information to Thompson's group home manager.

Thompson returned to KC's Sporting Goods on the appointed day, picked up his gun, and bought a box of blunt-nosed .38 ammunition. Before getting possession of the weapon, however, he had to complete a written questionnaire required by law. One of the questions gave him trouble: Had he been convicted of a felony or confined to a mental hospital? He first answered yes; after reflection, however, he marked out that answer and substituted no. The store clerk thought this unremarkable.

Both store workers then on duty thought Thompson a pleasant and gentle person. One clerk thought he was a college professor or physician. Thompson noted that the other worker looked depressed—as indeed she was. "Cheer up," he advised her, and smiled. "It's a nice day."

A few minutes later, Thompson walked into the personnel office at Metropolitan Hospital and resigned his 20-hour-per-week job. "I'm gonna be doing something else," he said.

THE MURDER

The next morning, Thompson rose at 5 a.m., as usual. He seemed unusually cheerful, and his vigorous whistling in the shower disturbed another resident, who stepped into the bathroom long enough to tell Thompson to "shut the goddamn up."

"Shit on you, man," Thompson responded, but he didn't seem particularly angry or upset by the encounter.

Showered and dressed, Thompson went downstairs and passed half an hour reading before going to the kitchen for breakfast. He seemed to have a hearty appetite, and the cook later described him as "giggly." Thompson cleared his place at the table and helped the cook clean and put away dishes.

Meanwhile, another of his roommates awakened. He noted Thompson's suitcase lying open on his bed, filled with clothes and surrounded by loose papers. Also scattered on the bed was about $30 in change and small currency. A small cardboard box labeled "Ammunition—50 rounds" also lay upon the bed, thus far unnoticed. Six shells were missing.

Thompson left the house at 8 a.m., saying he was bound for his job at Metro. He was back in the group home by 8:30, humming, whistling, and walking about. His apparent tardiness for work went unremarked in the bustle of the morning, but a social work technician noted at the time that he seemed "in a really good mood."

At 10 a.m., Thompson approached the social worker who served as supervisor of the home, and said he needed a ride to the mental health center. The supervisor telephoned Devon Hills, was told that Thompson was too late to make a scheduled appointment with Dr. Bettleman and was advised that he could still see a psychiatrist if he came right away.

The supervisor later reported that Thompson looked unusually happy when he drove him to the mental health center. He was smiling as he repeatedly adjusted the car radio in an unsuccessful search for a favorite station. At his destination, Thompson thanked the supervisor and exited the car. The last time the social worker saw him, Thompson was ambling up the paved walk in front of the center.

Inside the building, Thompson passed through the lobby and walked to the information desk. The receptionist heard him say something, but his tone was so low and indistinct that she couldn't understand him. She asked him twice to repeat what he had said.

"I'm Ray Thompson," he stated. "I'm here to see a doctor."

"Which doctor would you like to see?" the receptionist inquired.

"I don't remember his name," Thompson replied. "Just a doctor."

The receptionist consulted a schedule book, recorded Thompson's name on a contact card, and placed it beside those of others waiting for Bettleman. "If you'll take a seat," she said, "someone will see you when they're available."

Thompson turned and looked over the lobby for a moment, then took a seat beside Steven Sanger, another resident at his group home. Sanger asked him what he was doing at the center.

"I'm gonna see Dr. Clayton," he replied. Thompson seemed unaware that John Clayton, his primary therapist, was on vacation.

Sanger was also unaware of Clayton's absence. He remarked that Thompson was wearing his distinctive orange Metropolitan Hospital windbreaker and asked how his work was going.

"I'm gonna get a job here, talking to you people," Thompson answered. Sanger later reported that Thompson sounded angry or upset. "People here are different. They've got murderers and rapists. I can trust 'em."

The conversation was interrupted when Alan Woods came into the lobby carrying Sanger's file. "Your turn, Steven," he said. Woods and Sanger left the lobby together and turned into the hallway leading to Woods' office.

A minute later, Thompson left the lobby unnoticed and walked down the same passage. He quickly came to Woods' door, pushed it open, and stepped into the room. Thompson looked at the psychiatrist, seemingly ignoring Sanger's presence.

"Are you a psychiatrist?" he asked in an even, apparently calm voice.

"Yes, I am," Woods replied. He seemed about to add something, but Thompson interrupted.

"Then, I've got something for you," he stated, and drew the pistol from the waistband of his pants. He fired the weapon in Woods' direction again and again, until the hammer clicked on emptied chambers. Then he pushed the gun inside his belt and stared at his victim for a moment. "Our Father," he whispered in a prayer-like tone. "I can't believe I did that." His voice sounded calm and peaceful after the explosions from the .38. Thompson left the office and walked slowly down the hall. He passed the receptionist and clients in the lobby, who still were unaware that anything was amiss, and left the building.

A group home resident was on the walkway in front of the center on his way to the detached building housing the agency's day hospital program. Spying Thompson, he approached him, calling, "How ya doin', Ray?" and playfully swinging his fist at Thompson's arm.

"Hey, don't do that," Thompson replied, backing away. "I've had enough violence today."

Inside the center, Sanger meanwhile had rushed to Woods' side. Four bullets had struck the psychiatrist in the head and shoulder, splattering blood, bone, and bits of brain across the floor and wall behind him. Unknown to Sanger, another two shells had passed completely through the plasterboard wall and narrowly missed a psychologist and her client in the adjoining room.

As loud as the shots sounded in the confined space of Woods' office, few people in the building knew that a gun had been fired. Most who had heard the noise assumed that an angry patient was pounding on a wall or banging on a table with a metal ruler, a common event in any mental health center. Others thought the sounds came from the heating ductwork or some outside construction project. Those who recognized the gunfire were those in the immediate vicinity of Woods' office. Except for the psychologist and her patient, now hiding behind her desk, no one knew from where the shots came.

Ignorance changed to horror when Sanger rushed from the room and into the lobby. "Doctor Woods is dead," he blurted to the incredulous receptionist. "Ray Thompson just killed him." He pointed to the orange-jacketed figure walking along a sidewalk in front of the building.

When the painful truth of Sanger's statement was verified, the city police were called and word of the tragedy passed among the center staff. A few minutes later, a social worker in the day hospital approached one of the first uniformed officers to arrive.

"I think you're looking for Ray Thompson," he said. "He's wearing a bright orange jacket. Right now, he's sitting in my day room."

Officers accompanied the social worker to the building adjoining the main mental health center. A sergeant entered the day room to find Thompson sitting by himself on a sofa. He seemed peaceful, almost serene in contrast to the 15 to 20 clients milling about the room.

The sergeant had Thompson rise and lean against a wall and searched him for weapons. The pat-down revealed a .38-caliber revolver in his left front pants pocket. She handcuffed him and read him his Miranda rights.

"I refuse to say anything," Thompson replied.

The officer wasn't fazed. "Did anybody get hurt in the doctor's office?" she asked.

"It was an it," Thompson answered. "Is it dead?"

"Yes."

Thompson smiled. "I refuse to say anything," he repeated.

Thompson subsequently spent several months at Central State Hospital incompetent for trial. In the murder trial that followed his return to Lexington, the defense accepted the contention that Thompson had indeed killed Alan Woods. From the beginning, both sides focused on the defendant's mental state at the time of the offense. One after another, the people Thompson had encountered that day—the supervisor and cook at the group home, staff members and clients at the mental health center, and arresting officers—described Thompson as coherent and rational. No one reported the defendant discussing homicide, threats, persecution by psychiatrists, delusional ideations, or hallucinations.

Two psychiatrists and three psychologists were called as expert witnesses. Thompson's public defender pressed for suggestions of possible insanity during the commission of the murder. The prosecution, on the other hand, portrayed the defendant as a manipulator and malingerer trying to escape punishment by feigning mental illness.

The jury found Thompson guilty as charged of first degree murder. The defendant was subsequently sentenced to incarceration for the duration of his natural life. He is not eligible for parole.

Raymond Colette Thompson now resides at Mountain Dell State Prison. His conviction and sentence have not yet been appealed.

COULD THIS MURDER HAVE BEEN PREDICTED?

Most experienced psychologists have probably been verbally or physically threatened by clients. Inpatient involuntary psychiatric populations often include patients who refuse treatment, argue against their commitment status, accuse staff of conspiring against them, covertly or overtly refuse to take their medications, and taunt psychologists, psychiatrists, social workers, and especially ward personnel. An informal survey of one of the author's forensic populations indicated that about one out of three had threatened hospital workers during admission. Obviously, few such persons are later charged with homicide or attempted homicide of mental health providers. If all suspicious, guarded, paranoid schizophrenics with delusions of persecution and accompanying antisocial personality traits were predicted to attempt the murder of their therapists, the Type I error would be staggeringly high.

Could anything specific to Thompson's case have warned his care providers that he was likely to shoot a treatment professional? Perhaps. Thompson had a history of attempted and completed violence against persons. He had also at one time owned an impressive collection of firearms and continued to exhibit interest in guns after losing his own collection. He also seemed to be obsessed with the evils of psychotropics.

Basing her work upon the suicidal risk inventory of Hatton, Valente, and Rink,[1] sociologist Nancy Allen[2] has devised a simple inventory to aid in evaluating the likelihood of an individual committing homicide. She has emphasized that the application of any such assessment requires considerable caution and careful judgment. It should be noted that despite their obvious face validity, neither reliability nor predictive validity of Allen's schedule has been demonstrated. It does, however, seem to have considerable use as a starting point in evaluating homicidal risk. Of the 23 clinical characteristics Allen presents, Thompson was a high-risk candidate in 12 areas prior to the murder:

1. his past history indicated at least one early episode of extreme violence;
2. he had no significant others available to him;
3. he displayed an unstable life style;
4. he had a poor employment record;
5. he had long been considered self-isolating and withdrawn;
6. he had a considerable record of psychiatric hospitalization and a clearly negative appreciation of mental health services;
7. he appeared chronically moody;
8. his repeated aggressive behaviors had been recorded;
9. his poor impulse control was apparent;
10. his stress had historically led to socially unacceptable acting out;
11. he was apparently prone to reduced reality contact; and
12. he seemed unable or unwilling to use available resources to improve his condition in life.

In addition, just before the murder, Thompson displayed behavioral changes that could have indicated that violence of some sort was pending:

1. he stopped taking medications;
2. he quit his job;
3. he exhibited changes in mood, becoming unusually cheerful; and
4. he packed his bags.

These events would have signaled action had they been displayed by a depressed client with a history of self-destructive gestures. Most of us, however, are far more familiar with the precursors to suicide than the harbingers of murder. As a result, we probably attend less than we should to clues of impending homicide.

COULD THIS MURDER HAVE BEEN PREVENTED?

Assuming that it was possible to predict Thompson's threat to an unspecified mental health worker in a rather global fashion, could the murder have been prevented? Again, perhaps.

Although such a killing could certainly have been forestalled in theory, some practical applications would have required management methods common in correction facilities, but maybe inimical to community resources. Armed guards and metal detectors, once unknown beyond prison walls, are now regularly encountered at airports and courthouses. Security programs might have prevented Woods' murder at Devon Hills. They would not, however, have forestalled an attack on him at home. In addition, few private practitioners can afford such protection. Finally, these measures would seem out of place in some patient mental health programs.

An alternative to power and control approaches would require enhanced awareness of jeopardy and improved communications between and within agencies. A reasonable scenario would begin with Thompson's work supervisor being warned of his potential dangerousness. Then, when he quits his job following a period of declining productivity and attendance, the group home manager would be alerted. Thompson would be restricted to the residence, and a special joint conference would be held that very day. Thompson's behavioral changes would be discussed, and their disturbing pattern would unfold. Following an interview, Thompson, who would be restricted and closely observed in the day room, would be searched, as would his belongings and the home's public spaces. The gun, ammunition, or receipts would be found. Since possessing a firearm violates Thompson's release conditions, house rules, and state law, the police would be notified. The court would eventually determine whether Thompson would require commitment to a secure psychiatric facility, confinement in a penal institution, or return to a supervised community living arrangement.

IMPLICATIONS AND RECOMMENDATIONS

Alan Woods' murder and the events leading to it have a number of implications. While they may not be entirely novel, their direct connection to the security of mental health providers rarely has been made.

Mental Health Professionals

Psychologists and other mental health workers need to be aware that they may be targets for assassination. It is curious that the very persons with whom police and courts consult regarding dangerous mentally ill offenders seem so unprepared to predict, forestall, and protect themselves from murder. Given the severity of homicide as a social ill and personal threat, some sort of specialized training in recognizing precursors to homicide may be warranted.

Federal reports[3] indicate that 23,044 Americans were victims of murder and non-negligent manslaughter in 1980. That same year, 218 persons were murdered in New Orleans and 44 in our pseudonymous community of Lexington.[4] If current rates continue—and there is no reason to expect a precipitous decline—about a quarter of a million citizens will be killed by their fellows in this decade. These numbers argue for more professional involvement in determining precursors to homicide to identify at-risk offenders and victims and create early threat interventions.

Mental Health Agencies

Every analysis of intervention systems, social problems, and public or private tragedies seems to recommend improving communications. It cannot be stated with assurance that Alan Woods' life could have been saved by enhanced discourse across organizational boundaries and between personnel within individual organizations. But the question remains: would things have been different if a mental health professional had been aware of Thompson's background and his behavior immediately preceding the killing and had been able to properly assess the situation? Clues to a pending homicide existed, but were scattered across three years of records, reports, and observations, and distributed across several treatment programs. Obviously, care providers need to be better apprised of potential dangers and unexplained alterations in the behavior of their clients whose histories indicate a propensity for violence.

Thompson had very easy access to Woods' office, which raises another issue. Clinics and practitioners may need to review their accessibility. Some mental health centers, especially in urban areas, already have a single patient entrance, require staff escorts for clients in hallways, and employ security guards. Such stringent protection may be unnecessary in all programs and infeasible in some, but a careful evaluation of security requirements appears warranted.

Society

Most murders in this country are committed with handguns.[2,3] Despite this, the distribution of handguns is almost completely without restriction. Among the few regulations controlling firearms are prohibitions against their possession by ex-convicts, probationers, and persons who have been involuntarily committed to psychiatric care. These rules appear to be largely without teeth. Not only was Thompson violating the law when he purchased the pistol used in Woods' murder, he had difficulty completing the required form. He was nevertheless allowed to gain possession of a weapon, the sole purpose of which is to kill people. It would seem that discussions of the pros and cons of handgun legislation need to take into account the meaninglessness of present limited regulations. The wisdom of unrestricted access to handguns needs careful reconsideration.

CONCLUSION

From all accounts, Alan Woods' death was a tragedy of the first magnitude to his family, friends, patients, and co-workers. Perhaps by reviewing this and other episodes, similar calamities can be avoided in the future.

NOTES

1. Hatton, C. L., Valente, S., & Rink, A. (1976). *Suicide Assessment and Intervention.* New York: Appleton-Century Crofts.

2. Allen, N. H. (1980). *Homicide: Perspectives on Prevention.* New York: Human Services Press.

3. U. S. Department of Justice, Federal Bureau of Investigation (1981). *Crime in the United States, 1980.* Washington, DC: U. S. Government Printing Office.

4. Flanagan, T. J., & McLeod, M. (1983) (eds.), *Sourcebook of Criminal Justice Statistics—1982.* Washington, DC: U. S. Government Printing Office.

Chapter 3

Violence: The Psychiatric Patient

Kenneth Tardiff, M.D., M.P.H.

INTRODUCTION

Psychiatric patients are of particular interest to the public because of the fear generated by widespread media coverage of notorious murders committed by some of them. Yet these sensationalized murders may be the tip of the iceberg in terms of violence. Many psychiatric patients are now outside of institutions in the community secondary to deinstitutionalization policies. Many of these patients offend others in their communities by their antisocial behavior short of violence, such as cursing, being unkempt, and otherwise violating the norms of society. There is concern that psychiatric patients are more likely than the general population to be violent and commit crimes. There are conflicting studies about this point; some authors have found that psychiatric patients are at increased risk of engaging in violent and criminal activity, while others have argued that the prior criminal history of each psychiatric patient must be taken into account.[1] As we shall see, certain types of psychiatric patients pose greater risks of exhibiting violent behavior than other types.

Of more immediate concern is the safety of professionals working with psychiatric patients. There are a number of studies showing that assault may be an occupational hazard. Approximately 40 percent of psychiatrists have reported being assaulted at least once in their careers.[2,3] Another study found that 48 percent of psychiatric residents in a training program were assaulted at least once during the several years of their training.[4] Another study found that 24 percent of other mental health professionals in a number of disciplines reported being assaulted at least once in the previous year, but more psychiatrists (34 percent) than other mental health professionals reported being assaulted.[5]

In this chapter, I will review representative research on the frequency and patterns of violent behavior by psychiatric patients. I will discuss various aspects of the phenomenology of violence, particularly as it relates to etiology and management. It is important to recognize that for both etiology and treatment, consideration must be given to the social or environmental context in which the violent behavior occurs, as well as the psychological and biological characteristics of the patient. I will discuss the clinical management of the violent psychiatric patient in terms of emergency situations and long-term treatment as well as the administrative and legal implications of violence and its management.

RESEARCH ON VIOLENCE COMMITTED BY PSYCHIATRIC PATIENTS

Early systematic research beyond anecdotal reports on violence committed by psychiatric patients involved patients appearing for treatment in emergency rooms.[6] These patients manifested diffuse and extensive psychopathology with a predominance of personality disorders, some with evidence of seizure-like states or alcoholism. Yet many came to the emergency room on a voluntary basis seeking treatment. In general, later research involved patients with psychotic or severely incapacitating psychopathology. Some researchers have studied patients in treatment in specific diagnostic or age groups and have determined the characteristics of those who were violent and the frequency of their violent behavior. Four studies have examined small numbers of schizophrenic patients and have reported conflicting findings on rates of assaultive behavior and on whether certain subtypes of schizophrenia are associated with increased risk of assaultive behavior. Three of those studies found increased verbal or physical aggression in paranoid schizophrenics, while the fourth study found no increase of physical aggression in paranoid schizophrenics. Blackburn[7] examined 48 male schizophrenic patients and found that 63 percent of the paranoid schizophrenics and 24 percent of the nonparanoid schizophrenics had histories of aggressive behavior. Planasky and Johnson[8] found that 58 of 205 (29 percent) hospitalized male schizophrenic patients had made explicit verbal threats to kill or had attacked people. Again there was an increased likelihood of histories of homicidal threats or assaultive behavior in the paranoid schizophrenic group. Addad et al.[9] found that 53 of 116 (46 percent) schizophrenic patients had histories of previous criminal acts; paranoid schizophrenics, however, committed more crimes against persons, while nonparanoid schizophrenics were more likely to have committed nonviolent crimes. Shader et al.[10] examined 45 schizophrenic patients who had manifested physical aggression toward others; they found that schizoaffective schizophrenics were more likely than paranoid and other types of schizo-phrenics to have histories of physical aggression.

Fareta[11] assessed 438 patients from the ages of five to fifteen who were admitted to a state psychiatric hospital and found that 66 patients (15 percent), all twelve or older, had histories of serious violence, including homicides, sexual attacks, attacks or threats with deadly weapons, dangerous arson, and suicide attempts or threats. Those patients with histories of one or more of those behaviors were likely to be boys from minority groups, diagnosed as schizophrenic, with a low average intelligence quotient. Fareta was able to follow only 18 subjects for a period of 18 years; however, they did show a high degree of continued antisocial and criminal behavior.

Some researchers have sought to enlarge the scope of their surveys of violent behavior by using incident reports in hospitals; yet, there are two problems with the use of incident reports. First, there is under-reporting of violent episodes, which was demonstrated in a study by Lion, Snyder, and Merrill,[12] in which the actual occurrence of assault in a state hospital was five times that noted in routine incident reports. A second problem, statistical in nature, is the lack of accurate rates of violent behavior. Incident report studies have relied on the hospital census as denominator data, rather than on a clearly defined number of assessed patients. Thus, studies using incident reports have found differing rates of violence and conflicting patterns in terms of the characteristics of patients with a greater likelihood of violent behavior. In Sweden, Ekblom [13] found that only 34 inpatients out of a large number of patients were involved in reported violent incidents over a ten-year period. Kalogerakis[14] found only nine serious assaults in a six-year period at a municipal hospital and few violent incidents reported by five directors of state hospitals. Albee[15] examined all accident and incident reports for a two-year period at a large psychiatric institute and found that only 78 patients injured others during that time. Calculation of the rate of violent behavior was not possible, since there was no indication of the number of patients at risk. However, he did find an increased likelihood of violence by patients diagnosed as schizophrenic. Evenson, Altman, and Sletten[16] found 5,128 violent incidents, not only assaultive, involving 1,004 patients during a two-year period at a state hospital. Using the hospital census figures, they calculated that there were 99 incidents of assault per 1,000 patient years at risk. Schizophrenics were at low risk for all types of incidents, including assault, while neurotic patients, those with organic brain syndromes, and those with personality disorders all had an increased risk of assaultive behavior. In addition, male patients and nonwhite patients had a greater risk of assaultive behavior than female and white patients.

Fottrell[17] examined incident reports at two large psychiatric hospitals and one small psychiatric unit in a general hospital. Although the study author used incident reports, he felt certain that there was no under-reporting of assaults. Although exact rates of assault could not be calculated, since it was not clear how many patients were at risk, he stated that there were few serious assaultive incidents in the hospitals. In all assaultive incidents, regardless of severity, there was a preponderance of young patients who manifested assaultive behavior. Schizophrenia was the most common diagnosis among the offending patients, and the most common victims were staff members. Unfortunately, the proportion of patients with these demographic and clinical characteristics in the nonassaultive patient population was not determined. As a result of methodological limitations, it cannot be said that the young, female, or schizophrenic patients were actually overrepresented in the group of patients manifesting assaultive behavior in hospital.

Two studies attempted to assess more directly the occurrence of aggressive thoughts or action in psychiatric inpatients. Hagen, Mikolajczak, and Wright[18] asked 60 patients who were admitted consecutively to a private psychiatric hospital about their violent feelings or actions. They found that although the frequency of hostile or self-destructive feelings was high, the frequency of violent actions was rare. Benezech, Bourgeois, and Yesavage[19] reviewed the charts of 547 patients in a French hospital for the criminally insane and found that 47 percent of the patients had committed criminal acts against persons, especially assault or murder. Patients with psychotic disorders were more likely to have committed crimes against persons, while those with personality disorders were more likely to have committed criminal acts involving property.

The previous studies of the frequency and patterns of violence among psychiatric patients have not been broad enough in terms of diagnosis or have relied on incident reports. I will present the results of three of my studies that assessed the occurrence of assaultive behavior by patients just before admission to various types of psychiatric hospitals and by patients who had been in state hospitals for long periods of time.

The first study[20] looked at all patients admitted to public hospitals on Long Island during a one-year period. The source of data was the routinely computerized information from the New York State Department of Mental Hygiene. This data is collected for each patient on admission to a hospital or shortly thereafter. There were 594 (11.4 percent) male patients and 326 (7.9 percent) female patients who manifested assaultive behavior at the time of, or just prior to, admission to a hospital. Thus, assaultive behavior was more likely among male patients. The rest of the analysis was stratified by sex, the expectation being that violence may be expressed differently by male and female patients.

For both men and women, there was increased assaultive behavior in the young and among those 65 and older. In both sexes, there was an increased likelihood of assault by nonwhite patients at the high school educational level. For those above or below the high school level, however, there was no statistically significant association between race and rates of assaultive behavior. Marital status of patients was analyzed for those twenty-five or older. Both men and women who were assaultive were more likely to have never been married or to be widowed.

Primary psychiatric diagnosis was related to the occurrence of assaultive behavior. For both sexes, patients who had been assaultive were overrepresented in the diagnoses of organic mental disorders, paranoid schizophrenia, and "other diagnoses, predominantly personality disorders." Patients with alcohol or drug abuse as primary diagnoses were less likely to have manifested assaultive behavior. Schizophrenia, both paranoid and nonparanoid, was associated with increased assaultive behavior for male patients, while only nonparanoid schizophrenia was associated with assault by female patients. Men who were assaultive were twice as likely to have suicidal tendencies as men who were not assaultive. There was no association between assaultive behavior and suicide for female patients. There were no statistically significant relationships between assault and a history of seizures or whether the index admission was the first lifetime admission as opposed to a readmission controlling for the age of the patient. Assaultive patients were less likely to have received private psychiatric care in the past; however, they were more likely to have been incarcerated in the past. Assaultive patients were more likely to have been referred to the hospital by the police or courts.

The second study[21] looked at all patients admitted during a one-and-a-half-year period to the inpatient units of two private psychiatric hospitals in New York, one admitting only voluntary patients and the other admitting both involuntary and voluntary patients. In each hospital, one research assistant reviewed the completed hospital records for all patients admitted during the study period. The research assistants had experience in psychiatric nursing or clinical psychology. The data was recorded on structured work sheets.

There were 30 (9.8 percent) male and 28 (5.9 percent) female patients who were assaultive prior to admission to the voluntary private hospital, and 65 (15.5 percent) male and 42 (10.5 percent) female patients who were assaultive prior to admission to the involuntary private hospital. In general, the targets of the pre-admission assaults by patients placed in both hospitals were predominantly family members other than children or spouses and people outside of the family. There were fewer statistically significant relationships between assault and characteristics of patients at the hospital admitting only voluntary patients. However, the trend and pattern of assaultive behavior were consistent in the two hospitals. For both sexes, assaultive patients were more likely to be twenty years of age and younger, while for women only, those sixty-five and older were more likely to be assaultive than those twenty-one to sixty-four. Assaultive patients were more likely to be in the paranoid and nonparanoid schizophrenic and manic categories, and for female patients only, there was an association between assaultiveness and organic mental disorders. At neither hospital were there differences in terms of race or marital status and assaultive behavior.

At both hospitals, patients with histories of assault prior to admission were more likely than other patients to be placed in seclusion rooms during their hospital stays. At the voluntary private hospital, 43 percent of the male and 32 percent of the female assaultive patients had been placed in seclusion. This was approximately 2.5 times the frequency for nonassaultive patients at that hospital. At the involuntary private psychiatric hospital, 34 percent of the male and 43 percent of the female assaultive patients had been placed in seclusion. This was more than two times the frequency for nonassaultive patients at that hospital. Physical restraints were used very rarely at both hospitals. There were no differences between assaultive and nonassaultive patients in terms of the rate at which they experienced procedures to evaluate organicity, namely the use of electroencephalography, skull x-rays, psychological testing, or neurological consultations. However, female assaultive patients at the involuntary hospital did have a greater proportion of CAT scans, which is consistent with the increased frequency of organic mental disorders among female patients at that hospital. As in the other admission study, there was no association between alcohol problems and a history of assaultive behavior.

In comparing these studies of patients admitted to public versus private psychiatric hospitals, one is struck with the similarity in the rates of assaultive behavior, particularly at the private hospital admitting involuntary patients. Furthermore, the characteristics of patients with a greater likelihood of assault were generally similar for public and private hospitals in that assaultive patients were more likely to be men and in the younger age groups, although for both public and private hospitals, women over the age of sixty-five manifested increased rates of assaultive behavior compared to women in the middle age ranges, probably relative to organic mental disorders. Organicity, including seizures, did not appear to be associated with assaultive behavior among patients admitted to either public or private hospitals. As we will see in the next study, this was not the case among patients residing in state hospitals for long periods of time.

Craig[22] basically duplicated my first study by analyzing admission data for 876 patients admitted to state hospitals in a single county in New York in a retrospective study using data collected from August 1975 to July 1976. He found that 11 percent of patients hospitalized during the study period demonstrated assaultive behavior just before admission. Male schizophrenic patients, patients with other diagnoses, and patients with organic brain ʒyndromes showed significantly more assaultive behavior than patients in the diagnostic categories of depression, mania, or alcohol abuse. The rate and diagnostic differences between assaultive and nonassaultive patients are similar to those found in my admission studies. With stratification by diagnosis, there was a lack of statistically significant associations between the age, sex, and race of the patients and the presence of assaultive behavior. He concluded that the nature of the underlying psychopathology is the prime link to assaultive behavior and that other characteristics of patients are related to diagnoses. This is a point of disagreement, since I believe age and sex in addition to diagnosis are related to assault outside of the hospital.

The last study was a survey of all patients residing in two large state hospitals in New York.[23] All patients residing in these hospitals for longer than one month were included in the survey except for those in special treatment units for alcoholism or mental retardation and those under 17 years of age. (Patients who were in the hospital for less than one month were excluded, since we were not interested in the acute phase of illnesses, which had been covered in the admission studies.) The surveyors were experienced staff members, predominantly nurses in the hospitals, but they did not assess patients on the wards in which they worked. Surveyors participated in training workshops to familiarize themselves with a manual of operational definitions for items on the survey instrument. To assess a patient, the surveyor interviewed the patient and the staff members working with the patient and reviewed the medical record.

The instrument for this survey was a revised version of that used in a previous inpatient survey of the psychological and physical status of mental patients.[24] The instrument in the revised inpatient survey included a clear definition of assault, specifying that assault was physically directed toward persons, and indicated a time frame during which the assault occurred; namely, that it occurred at least once within the hospital in the three months preceding the survey. Of the 5,164 patients, there were 186 (3.6 percent) male patients and 198 (3.8 percent) female patients who physically assaulted other persons at least once in the preceding three months. Thus, there was no difference between men and women in terms of the proportion of patients who were assaultive in the hospital. Approximately two-thirds of the most recent assaults occurred within the month preceding the survey. Assaultive patients were more likely than nonassaultive patients to be younger than forty-four and were especially overrepresented in the 17-34 age groups. The subgroup of male patients from seventeen to thirty-four years of age had a particularly high frequency of assault, five times that of the general patient population. Assaultive patients were more likely to have been in hospital for a shorter period of time than nonassaultive patients; however, this still involved periods of time in terms of years. For both sexes, assaultive patients were overrepresented in the diagnostic categories of nonparanoid schizophrenia, psychotic organic brain syndrome, other nonpsychotic disorders, and mental retardation. Surprisingly, assaultive patients were underrepresented in the category of paranoid schizophrenia. Of those patients who were psychotic, assaultive patients were more severely impaired in terms of delusions, hallucinations, and bizarre and antisocial behavior.

Another clinical difference was the increased likelihood of seizure disorders (21 percent) as a current problem for both male and female assaultive patients, more than twice that for nonassaultive patients. Further analysis showed that only primary psychiatric diagnosis was a factor in differentiating assaultive patients with seizures from those without seizures. Assaultive patients with seizures were more likely to be diagnosed with psychotic organic brain syndromes, mental retardation, or other nonpsychotic disorders. In only one-fourth of the patients with seizures and psychotic organic brain syndromes was the latter associated with epilepsy alone; in the rest it was associated with cerebral arteriosclerosis, senile dementia, or alcohol.

Interestingly, assaultive patients were more likely than nonassaultive patients to cry and express feelings of depression. A further indication that assaultive patients were more prone to have depressive symptomatology lies in the finding that male assaultive patients were three times more likely and female assaultive patients were more than four times more likely than nonassaultive patients to have attempted suicide at least once.

As expected, assaultive patients were more likely than nonassaultive patients to have received, at least once in the preceding month, emergency administration of medication, to have been placed in seclusion, in a strait-jacket or in other physical restraints, and to have received one-to-one or constant observation on the ward in order to control their dangerous behavior.[25] Assaultive patients in the youngest age groups were almost twice as likely to have received all types of control measures. Assaultive patients in the diagnostic categories of mental retardation and other nonpsychotic disorders had a greater likelihood of receiving all three controls, while nonparanoid schizophrenics were more likely to have received only emergency medication and one-to-one supervision. Although the other diagnostic groups were not increased relative to the diagnostic categories of mental retardation, nonpsychotic disorders, and nonparanoid schizophrenia, the overall percentages of assaultive patients receiving emergency medication (40 percent), one-to-one supervision (27 percent), and seclusion or physical restraints (17 percent) were substantial and no doubt represent considerable staff effort and time in managing dangerous behavior on the wards.

For the 384 patients with histories of assault in the hospital, the types and doses of medications received on a daily basis were categorized.[26] Drug combinations were infrequent and predominantly involved anticonvulsants and neuroleptics. Approximately three-fourths of the patients were given neuroleptics routinely, usually as the only drug, but occasionally in combination with anticonvulsants. Those neuroleptic drugs used most frequently alone were haloperidol, chlorpromazine, thioridizine, and thiothixene. Few patients were on multiple neuroleptics or tricyclic antidepressants, the latter usually given with neuroleptics. Two patients were on lithium carbonate with neuroleptics. Only 53 (13.8 percent) of the assaultive patients received no daily psychoactive medication.

Two characteristics of the patients were related at a statistically significant level to the type of medication the patients received routinely. First, younger patients, especially those in the seventeen to thirty-four age group (90 percent), were more likely to be on neuroleptic drugs, while those patients sixty-five or older (26 percent) were more likely than patients in other age groups to be receiving no psychiatric medication on a daily basis.

Second, diagnosis was related to the type of medication prescribed. As expected, schizophrenics were treated with neuroleptics; however, patients with diagnoses of mental retardation and other nonpsychotic disorders were also more likely than other patients to be treated on a daily basis with neuroleptics. Even though patients with psychotic organic brain syndrome were proportionately more likely than those in other diagnostic groups to be on no routine medication, 65 percent of these patients were on neuroleptics, with or without other medications. Length of stay in the hospital, sex, and race were not associated at a statistically significant level with the type of medication given routinely.

In addition, patients were classified as receiving high, regular, or low daily doses of medication. The suggested daily dose in the *AMA Drug Evaluations*[27] was considered to be a regular dose. Those patients receiving daily doses below this were classified as being in the low category, and those above the suggested dose were in the high category. In cases where there were combinations of anticonvulsants and neuroleptics with different dose categories for each drug, the dose of the neuroleptic was used for classification. There were seven cases excluded from this portion of the analysis because they could not be classified in the low-, regular-, or high-dose categories since they were receiving multiple neuroleptics or neuroleptics and antidepressants in differing dose categories.

Of the assaultive patients on medication, 64 percent were on daily doses within the ranges suggested by the *AMA Drug Evaluations*, while 20 percent were on higher doses, and 16 percent were on doses lower than the suggested ranges. Younger patients were on higher doses, and those sixty-five and older were on lower doses. Men were on higher doses than women. In terms of diagnoses, nonparanoid schizophrenics were on higher doses, while patients with psychotic organic brain syndromes or depression were on lower daily doses. Daily doses of neuroleptics were not related to the presence of seizure disorders, thus indicating that doses of neuroleptics given with anticonvulsants were not lowered for patients with seizure disorders, despite evidence that they can lower the seizure threshold.[28] Assaultive patients on high doses of medications were more likely than those on lower doses to have been given emergency medication, to have been put in seclusion or physical restraints, and to require one-to-one supervision in the month preceding the survey to control dangerous behavior.

The surveyors placed each patient at one of four levels in terms of mental status and treatment needed. For analysis of this data, only patients who had been in hospital for longer than three months were included, since it would be more likely that they had stabilized to a large degree and would not be in the acute phase of illness.[29] As expected, seven percent of male patients and four percent of female patients with histories of at least one assaultive episode were placed at level one, that is, as still dangerous to others at the time of the survey and requiring a highly secure psychiatric environment. Less than one percent of patients without histories of assault in the preceding three months were placed at that level. Patients with histories of assault were three times more likely than nonassaultive patients to be placed at level two, that is, showing severe psychotic symptomatology at the time of the survey and requiring intensive psychiatric services in the inpatient unit. Although the proportion was greater for nonassaultive patients, most patients were placed at level three, indicating that psychiatric symptoms had stabilized, but there was a continued need for inpatient treatment. Last, only 13 percent of male patients and 12 percent of female patients with histories of assault were deemed appropriate for community placement. Patients without histories of assault were twice as likely to be appropriate for community placement.

The rest of the analysis focused on the 359 patients in hospital for longer than three months with histories of assault; it determined which assaultive patients were deemed appropriate for community placement and which needed various levels of inpatient supervision. Only age and diagnosis were related to the assignment of assaultive patients to levels of supervision. Those assaultive patients assigned to level one—that is, those requiring a secure environment for current behavior dangerous to others, were more likely to be under thirty-four and to have a primary psychiatric diagnosis of mental retardation. Assaultive patients assigned to level two—that is, those needing intensive supervision for severe psychotic symptoms but not currently dangerous to others, were more likely to be under thirty-four and diagnosed as having schizophrenia of a type other than paranoid. Assaultive patients assigned to level three, who had stabilized in terms of symptoms but who were not appropriate for community placement, were older than sixty-five and overrepresented in the psychotic organic brain syndrome and other nonpsychotic disorder diagnostic categories. Assaultive patients assigned to level four—those appropriate for community placement—were likely to be in the thirty-four to sixty-four-year age group and in the diagnostic categories of paranoid schizophrenia and depression.

In conclusion, my surveys indicate that rates of assaultive behavior are higher among psychiatric patients just before, or at the time of, admission to hospitals—that is, outside of hospitals. Interestingly, the rates for private and public hospitals were similar, and they were higher than rates for patients who were residing in state hospitals for long periods of time. Rates of assaultive behavior for patients in the admission studies were found to be higher for males than for females. For patients residing in hospitals for long periods of time, females were just as likely as males to manifest assaultive behavior. One may speculate that the sex is less of a factor in aggressive behavior for patients who have resided in hospitals for long periods of time. In all of the studies, patients in the youngest age groups were more likely to manifest assaultive behavior. The only exception was for those patients older than sixty-five, and it was apparent that this was associated with organic deficits.

In terms of diagnosis, schizophrenics, both nonparanoid and paranoid, were more likely to have been assaultive just before, or at the time of, admission to the hospital. Among patients residing in hospitals for long periods of time, nonparanoid schizophrenics had greater rates of assault than paranoid schizophrenics. One may speculate that paranoid schizophrenics, once admitted to a hospital, are more able to control their actions, even though delusions or other psychopathology continue to exist. In addition, they may be more amenable to treatment and discharge into the community. However, once discharged, there is a possibility that paranoid schizophrenics are more likely to discontinue their medication and manifest a reemergence of delusional thinking, a loss of control, and an increased likelihood of subsequent assaultive behavior.

There was evidence that organic mental disorders and mental retardation are associated with increased rates of assaultive behavior, and, for those assaultive patients continuing to reside in hospitals, seizures and other organic deficits may play an important role in assaultive behavior. In all types of hospitals, emergency control measures were used frequently for assaultive patients; however, they differed depending upon the type of hospital. In public hospitals, both seclusion and restraint were frequently used, whereas in private hospitals, only seclusion was used to manage assaultive behavior. Routine medications for assaultive inpatients appeared to be appropriate in terms of type and dosage, except in state hospitals, where mentally retarded patients were on routine neuroleptic medication. This is problematic, since there is a definite risk of irreversible side effects with long-term use of neuroleptic medication and evidence that these medications may decrease learning in mentally retarded patients.[30]

Types of Violence

Violence can be described and classified along a number of parameters. First, the target of violence can be indicated, for example, persons versus objects in the environment. Furthermore, if the targets of violence are persons, the type of person should be specified; for example, the characteristics of the staff member or the family member as well as the reason, if any, need to be stated. A male staff member attacked by a male patient with pseudohomosexual panic or a family member attacked secondary to a patient having paranoid delusional thinking involving that family member represent different bases for the violent behavior. Even patients with low levels of intellectual functioning may have underlying psychodynamics related to violent episodes, such as the mentally retarded adolescent who pulls only the hair of the female nursing staff.

Along different parameters, violence toward persons or the physical environment may be the result of deliberate behavior, as in the case of those with antisocial or other personality disorders or paranoid delusional thinking, or as a result of disorganized, impulsive, nondeliberate behavior, as in the case of patients with organic brain syndromes, mania, or nonparanoid schizophrenia. Another dimension by which violence may be described is the degree of injury or damage. Obviously, violence resulting in broken bones, lacerations, the loss of an eye or even the life of a victim, or massive destruction of a ward by arson would have different management and prevention implications than violence resulting in no permanent physical injury or in minor property damage. Along similar lines, violence such as assault against or murder of a famous person or involvement in a highly publicized murder will have different treatment implications, mainly in terms of the reaction of staff members and patients and the degree of security measures in the inpatient setting. An exception in which minor violence requires major measures is when minor violence has preceded more serious violence by a patient. Familiar with a particular patient, staff members may rely on past violent episodes in terms of patterns of verbal and nonverbal cues that have preceded more serious violent episodes in the past. If the staff can predict with confidence that more serious violent behavior will follow minor violent behavior or verbal aggression, then the more restrictive control mechanisms—involuntary medication, seclusion, or restraint—may be indicated as preventive measures.

In terms of the management of a violent patient, especially in the emergency situation, the most important distinction in terms of type of violence involves whether the patients will respond to verbal communication with the clinicians and thus control themselves. Often, this involves an instant differential diagnosis on the part of the clinician. The patients least likely to respond to verbal communication are those with diagnoses of mania, schizophrenia, or organic mental disorders. Patients with personality disorders or other nonpsychotic diagnoses, without the heavy influence of alcohol or drugs, are more likely to respond to verbal interchange with the clinician. The management of patients in three distinct groups—those with organic brain disorders, functional pyschoses, and personality or other nonpsychotic disorders—will be discussed later in the chapter. Suffice it to say that violence may result from organic mental disorders associated with epilepsy, infections, hypoxia, and other causes of deliria; brain tumors; dementia; and mental retardation. The functional psychoses of schizophrenia and manic-depressive disorders are clear-cut, and violence by patients thus diagnosed may be either deliberate or impulsive and disorganized. Violence related to personality disorders may be a lifelong pattern of discrete episodes often associated with a history of poor impulse control. On the other hand, violent episodes may be infrequent yet serious occurrences for an individual who is overcontrolled, rigid, and isolated from society.

Understanding the Sources of Violence

To understand the sources of violence as well as its management, it is necessary to consider the biological, psychological, and social spheres. In each violent person, there is a biological substrate for violence, whether it is basic neurophysiological mechanisms in the brain or unique influences for the particular person, such as genetic inheritance, low intelligence, hormones, gross organic brain lesions, or other major psychiatric disorders. This biological substrate is tempered by learning, modeling, and the influences of family, peers, and society that result in the psychological profile of the individual. A violent episode is triggered by such factors as stress; frustration; economic considerations; the physical environment, including heat, crowding, and noise; and conflict with other individuals, such as family members, friends, or staff members.

Thus, the environment of the treatment setting is just as important as the psychological and biological characteristics of the psychiatric patient in producing or preventing a violent episode. Patients must have the opportunity to participate in their environment and to interact with staff members and other patients. It is necessary to design individual treatment programs that fit the tolerance of, and need for, social stimulation of patients with various disorders. Recreational materials and structured activities should be available. Staff members should realize that some patients need assistance to make use of recreational and rehabilitative activities. Active outreach by staff members is necessary to ensure that patients are engaged in appropriate levels of activities, otherwise patients regress and become isolated and eventually violent.

Rada[31] pointed out that violence on a general hospital or a psychiatric ward commonly expresses the patients' anger toward the staff, family, themselves, or their illnesses. Violence may be the result of poor communication between the physician and patient that has led to a lack of trust. Instead of striking out at the physician, patients may threaten or strike out against nurses, aides, or family members. Reestablishing lines of communication between the patient and the treating physician can often bring immediate relief to both patient and staff.

Lion[32] has described a number of countertransference problems that can occur in physicians and other treatment personnel. They may find themselves irrationally frightened of or inappropriately angry with patients because of their own past experiences with violence. A violent patient may evoke a positive countertransference reaction that interferes with treatment. A physician with personal conflicts regarding aggression may overidentify with violent patients or act out personal hostilities with the patient. Another mechanism with which to handle conflicts about violence is denial. This is very dangerous, since it may interfere with clinicians' ability to take proper precautions with their safety and the safety of others. Countertransference reactions of staff members produce a number of interesting, and at times counterproductive, patterns in inpatient units. In staff conferences, differences in how staff view violent patients' dangerousness may polarize meetings and produce conflict in the inpatient unit. In summary, the interaction of the violent patient with the physical and psychodynamic factors in the treatment setting must be observed and altered to minimize or prevent violence by psychiatric patients.

Management of the Violent Psychiatric Patient

Management is divided into emergency management of violent episodes and long-term treatment of violent patients. Above all, the patient must be in control while speaking with the clinician through self-control or through external physical controls, usually involuntary in nature. In his monograph, Lion[33] describes the typical emergency situation the clinician encounters in which the patient who is violent or was recently violent is found surrounded by staff members, family members, other patients, and perhaps security police in the hospital. He states that there is often a vicious cycle: a crowd struggles with the patient, which in turn increases resistance and violence by the patient. The ideal condition for interrupting this cycle is for the patient to be alone with the clinician. As previously mentioned, rapid diagnosis and decision making by the clinician must take place concerning whether the ideal condition is possible. The main question is whether the patient is amenable to verbal intervention as opposed to physical control.

The clinician is wise to exercise caution and avoid presenting a facade of bravado. If clinicians feel more comfortable initially having others around them with the violent patient, then they should not see the patient alone. It is important for the clinician to be comfortable with the violent patient so that a sense of security and calm competence can be conveyed.

The setting in which the patient is seen by the clinician will vary in terms of the degree of restrictiveness. This ranges from having the patient in physical restraints, to having the patient in an interview room with the clinician and attendants, to having the patient in an interview room alone with the clinician with the door either open or closed.

First, we will consider the most extreme situation in which the patient is violent, psychotic, and/or not amenable to verbal communication. Often, this patient must be physically restrained if only to be injected with medication. Recently, guidelines for the use of seclusion and restraint have been published.[34] They will be summarized here. Adequate manpower must be available, consisting of at least one person for each limb and another person who serves as the leader of the restraint procedure. Action by the staff must be rapid and must proceed without hesitation or further attempts at verbal communication with the patient. Implementation of restraint places the staff and patient at risk of injury; thus, it is necessary that facilities have written guidelines and that the procedure be rehearsed, observed, and critiqued as well as reviewed by the legal staff of the hospital. Efforts should be made to avoid humiliation of the patient and to preserve the appearance of routine and order throughout the procedure.

At a predetermined signal from the restraint leader, each staff member seizes and controls the movement of one extremity. The patient is brought to the ground with a backward movement, and each limb is restrained. The restraint leader controls the patient's head to prevent biting. In regard to the safety of the staff, potentially dangerous items such as jewelry or glasses should be removed before beginning the restraint procedure. In regard to the safety of the patient, certain techniques are not permissible, such as bending a joint beyond or contrary to its normal range of motion. Obviously, sitting on the patient, pulling the patient's hair, choking, hitting, or pinching is prohibited, as are words, acts, or gestures showing disrespect or lack of concern on the part of the staff. The primary therapist is best not involved physically in the restraint episode, since this may be a barrier to future verbal intervention with the patient.

Once the patient is controlled, mechanical restraints as indicated in the hospital's guidelines may be applied. In addition, or instead, the patient may be injected with the appropriate medication and/or placed in a seclusion room. Although the use of medication in the emergency situation will be discussed later, I should say a few words about the decision to use one or more alternatives, namely mechanical restraint, seclusion, and involuntary medication. The decision is strictly a clinical one and the issue should not be seen as a question of which alternative is more or less restrictive legally. Restraints may be used if the etiology of the violence is unknown, as in an organic mental disorder where one would not want to use medication. Restraint alone may be preferable to seclusion if it is feared that the patients would mutilate themselves or the condition would worsen with sensory isolation. Caution should be exercised in the use of medication in elderly patients whose medical conditions contraindicate their use. Seclusion may not be possible if the patient's unstable medical condition resulting from infection, cardiac illness, metabolic disorders, or other problems requires close monitoring and the physical proximity of staff. Patients for whom seclusion may be contraindicated include those who have experienced a paradoxical reaction to phenothiazine medication, those who have taken overdoses and require close monitoring, and, in situations where seclusion rooms are hot on summer days, patients on phenothiazines, which impair thermal regulation. In addition to being unpleasant if used over long periods of time, physical restraint may result in circulatory obstruction or, if the patients are lying on their backs, aspiration. Obviously, such patients in restraints must be monitored very closely.

Seclusion may be preferable in cases where prolonged restraint is to be avoided and in cases where patients may actually benefit from decreased sensory stimulation. Medication may be preferred to restraint or prolonged seclusion in cases of patients who would benefit from the direct action of medication, for example, neuroleptic medication for paranoid schizophrenics who are violent because of delusional thinking and have not been taking prescribed oral neuroleptic medication. On the other hand, the use of repetitive medication to control dangerous behavior in the mentally retarded patient would not be as desirable as using seclusion or restraint first. Last, seclusion may not be preferable for patients who manifest violent behavior as a means of isolating themselves from the rest of the ward milieu. Restraint and seclusion are usually implemented by nursing and other professional staff members in emergency situations, but they do require a physician's review and order for continuation. The physician should be notified as soon as possible, preferably within the hour. For the first episode of restraint or seclusion, the physician should see the patient, usually within three hours and preferably within one hour after the beginning of the restraint or seclusion episode. When notified by telephone, physicians should indicate their approval pending personal examination of the patients. For each subsequent restraint or seclusion episode for those patients, a physician is to be notified within the hour. However, the physician will exercise professional judgment as to whether a visit is necessary and will indicate any special precautions that must be taken or monitoring that must be done by nursing or other professional staff members.

The physician is to see a restrained or secluded patient as frequently as necessary to monitor any changes in the patient's physical or mental status. The frequency of these visits may vary; however, a minimum of two visits a day, approximately 12 hours apart, seems reasonable. Obviously, some patients will require more frequent visits, including those with concurrent medical problems, organic brain syndromes, such as those related to drugs or alcohol, and those at risk for hyperthermia.

A physician's order is generally valid for 12 hours. The physician should examine the patient and document in the patient's record the justification for continued seclusion or restraint.

During the period of time patients are in seclusion or restraints, observations regarding their behavior should be made every 15 minutes by members of the nursing staff. Such observations may be made by simply looking through the observation glass window of the seclusion room if opening the seclusion room door would place the nursing staff member at risk for injury. Previously agitated patients in seclusion or those who have received psychotropic medication in addition to being placed in seclusion should be visited no less than every two hours. These observations assure the safety of the patient and will enable the staff to evaluate the patient for eventual removal from seclusion. The basic needs of a patient in seclusion and restraint should be attended to, including toileting, meals, and proper administration of fluids. Proper precautions should be taken to ensure the safety of staff members as well as patients; for example, eating utensils should be blunt to prevent them from being used as weapons.

The patient is removed from seclusion or restraint after a series of observations of self-control and ability and willingness to follow instructions of the staff. After each episode of seclusion and restraint, the staff should discuss the episode in terms of technique to allow the release of tensions from staff members. In addition, the episode should be openly discussed among patients to allay fears associated with violence and staff use of force. Last, once the patient is removed from seclusion and restraint and in control of personal actions, the violent episode and the use of seclusion and restraint should be discussed with the individual in an effort to deal with the psychological impact on the patient and to prevent subsequent violent episodes.

Once the patient is in restraints or has re-established personal control, the clinician must determine whether there is an organic mental disorder, and if so, treat the etiology of the disorder. Although a discussion of the types of organic disorders is beyond the scope of this chapter, I will briefly consider a few types associated with violence. Rada[31] has found that toxic reactions to illicit drugs such as phencyclidine, LSD, barbiturates, amphetamines, and cocaine are common causes of violence in the emergency room. Violence may be associated with alcohol detoxification or withdrawal in states such as delirium tremens and alcohol hallucinosis. Other organic causes of violence include electrolyte imbalances, anoxia, and any other underlying cause of delirious states.

If organic brain syndrome has been ruled out and it appears the violent patient is schizophrenic or manic, then neuroleptic medication is indicated. In this situation, intramuscular medication is usually necessary, unless the patient has regained control and will voluntarily take oral medication. In a process called rapid neuroleptization, a drug such as haloperidol is given intramuscularly in doses of 2.5 to 10 mg every 30 minutes until the violent behavior is controlled. Donlon[35] has found that dosages up to 100 mg in 24 hours have been safe and effective. Again, blood pressure, pulse, rhythm, respiration, and level of consciousness must be carefully monitored, and a clinician must be equipped to manage any problems as they develop.

If the patient is not psychotic but is actively violent, barbiturates or diazepam should be considered. Tupin[36] prefers slow intravenous administration of either type of drug, since responses to intramuscular or oral administration are slow and erratic. He recommends a 10 percent solution of sodium amobarbital administered at a rate of 0.5-1 mg per minute in doses of 200 to 500 mg or 5 to 10 mg of diazepam, given slowly and intravenously. With both medications, it is necessary to look for side effects, such as depressed respiration or hypotension, and be prepared to resuscitate the patient.

Should the clinician decide that patients can control themselves as in the case of those with nonpsychotic disorders, then interviews with the patients alone can proceed. An interview room needs to provide an easy exit and should not contain objects that could be used as weapons, such as letter openers, bookends, or paperweights. If a desk is present, it should be arranged so that it separates individuals to a greater extent than is usually the case. Decorative cushions may double as protective devices. Ideally, a buzzer or some other device to signal persons outside of the room of impending danger to the clinician is advisable. Lion[33] advises the clinician to ask security personnel, nurses, or family members to wait down the hall. He states that this spares physicians great embarrassment should they not be able to fulfill the fantasies that other people have about them, namely that they are omnipotent.

Once alone with the patient, the clinician sits down and asks the patient to do likewise. The clinician then attempts to acknowledge the patient's anger and hostility in a calm, gentle, and down-to-earth fashion. Patients are encouraged to verbally express their anger. Derogatory, judgmental, or other questions that attack the patient's self-esteem are avoided. When the patient begins to talk. the physician then inquires about whether the patient wishes to take oral medication if indicated.

In the evaluation of a patient's problem with violence in the outpatient setting or emergency room, a decision must be made about whether the patient should be hospitalized. This is a process analagous to the evaluation of suicide potential. Evaluation of the patient requires an assessment of the seriousness of the actual violent episode. With threats of violence, one must consider how well planned they are. A man who has well-formulated plans about how to kill his employer should be taken much more seriously than someone who makes vague threats about getting even or striking out. at others. As with evaluation of suicide potential, the availability of a means of inflicting injury, a weapon, for example, is to be considered. The role of the intended victims and their behavior in provoking violence should be considered if the patients are to be returned to their homes. Furthermore, the use of alcohol or drugs increases the likelihood of impulsive, serious, violent behavior. Certain demographic characteristics must be considered. Young patients are more likely to be violent then are older patients, and men more than women. A history of previous violence forebodes problems with violence, as does a history of parental violence. Last, the presence of delusions and psychosis necessitates hospitalization. In addition to considering a patient's potential for violence toward others, one must also consider the potential for suicide, since it is often associated with violence.

Subsequent long-term therapy aims to treat the underlying psychiatric disorder. In the case of an individual with an organic mental disorder, this is preceded by a complete evaluation including appropriate lab tests for metabolic disorders or drugs, as well as a thorough neurological examination and appropriate diagnostic radiologic procedures. The electroencephalogram examination, including sleep and nasopharyngeal leads, is indicated for a number of violent patients, even when there is no clear-cut evidence of a seizure disorder. Again, treatment of a violent patient with a seizure disorder is directed toward the underlying disorder, as is the treatment of violent patients with schizophrenia or mania. The standard procedures in the latter case use neuroleptics or lithium carbonate with appropriate psychosocial intervention once the psychosis is stabilized.

I would like to briefly discuss the long-term treatment of the nonpsychotic violent patient primarily with psychotherapeutic techniques. Lion and Madden have outlined principles of psychotherapeutic treatment of the violent patient.[33,37] First, in addition to outpatient visits, the patient should be instructed to use the emergency room during moments of stress and incipient violent behavior. The primary goal in the psychotherapy is to enable the patient to talk, rather than act. Violent patients have a limited ability to express such emotions as anger, envy, or frustration. Rather, they convert these emotions into actions. The therapist should aim to help the patient identify emotional states, particularly those that have preceded violent action in the past. The choice of individual, couple, family, or group psychotherapy should be tailored for the specific patient. Often, individual psychotherapy is not the ideal treatment for violent patients who have difficulty with intimacy. In addition, it may be wise to include a spouse or other family members who are involved, often as participants in the pattern of violence by the patient. Group psychotherapy with cotherapists provides an atmosphere of control as well as a sense of support, while at the same time allowing peer pressure and confrontation in a controlled setting. This form of psychotherapy provides an opportunity to socialize and places a premium, again, on verbal, rather than behavioral, expressions of stress and emotion. In summary, the patient must develop trust in the therapist, learn to use verbal means of expression, and identify those situations and warning signs that precede violent behavior.

REVIEW OF IMPLICATIONS

Research has shown that violence among psychiatric patients is a significant problem that must be managed by mental health professionals. There are indications that some patients are at a higher risk of becoming violent than others. Guidelines for the management of violent psychiatric patients must be developed by each institution, whether an outpatient or inpatient setting. These guidelines range from recommendations about protection of the staff to the opposite extreme, the proper use of control mechanisms, such as seclusion, restraint, and involuntary medication. Furthermore, these guidelines should be subject to review by the institution's legal representatives. Good clinical judgment takes precedence in the use of physical controls and this position is fully supported by the Supreme Court in the *Youngberg v. Romeo* decision[38] concerning seclusion and restraint. The implication of the recent Massachusetts State decision in *Mill v. Rogers*,[39] which limits the use of involuntary medication, is still unclear and may tip the balance toward the use of seclusion and restraint in the management of violence in emergency situations. In all cases, though, good clinical judgment forms the foundation of policy by individual institutions.

The clinician must be skilled in the immediate diagnosis of the violent psychiatric patient in the emergency situation in order to determine whether verbal intervention is possible or whether the use of external physical controls in indicated. The emergency and long-term pharmacologic management of the violent patient usually is based on the treatment of the underlying psychiatric disorder. As in other areas of psychiatry, it is necessary to use treatment modalities in the biological, psychological, and social spheres. The importance of ensuring a proper treatment environment for patients is as important as skill in the use of medication and psychotherapy. Staff training in all three modalities is essential in the management of violent psychiatric patients.

NOTES

1. J. Rabkin, "Criminal Behavior of Discharged Mental Patients: An Initial Appraisal of the Research," *Psychological Bulletin* 86 (1979): 1-27.

2. D. J. Madden, J. R. Lion, and M. W. Penna, "Assault on Psychiatrists by Patients," *American Journal of Psychiatry* 133 (1976): 422-425.

3. K. Tardiff and W. Maurice, "The Care of Violent Patients by Psychiatrists: A Tale of Two Cities," *Canadian Psychiatric Association Journal* 22 (1977): 83-86.

4. I. Ruben, G. Wolkon, and J. Yamamoto, "Physical Attacks on Psychiatric Residents by Patients," *Journal of Nervous and Mental Disease* 168 (1980): 243-245.

5. R. M. Whitman, B. B. Armao, and O. B. Dent, "Assault on the Therapist," *American Journal of Psychiatry* 133 (1976): 426-431.

6. J. R. Lion, G. Bach-y-Rita, and F. R. Ervin, "Violent Patients in the Emergency Room," *American Journal of Psychiatry* 125 (1969): 1706-1711.

7. R. Blackburn, "Emotionality, Extraversion and Aggression of Paranoid and Non-paranoid Schizophrenic Offenders," *British Journal of Psychiatry* 115 (1968): 1301-1302.

8. K. Planasky and R. Johnston, "Homicidal Aggression in Schizophrenic Men," *Acta Psychiatrica Scandanavica* 55 (1977): 65-73.

9. M. Addad et al., "Criminal Acts Among Schizophrenics in French Mental Hospitals," *Journal of Nervous and Mental Disease* 169 (1981): 289-293.

10. R. I. Shader et al., "Patterns of Violent Behavior Among Schizophrenic Inpatients," *Diseases of the Nervous System* 38 (1977): 13-67.

11. G. Fareta, "A Profile of Aggression from Adolescence to Adulthood: An 18 Year Follow-up of Psychiatrically Disturbed and Violent Adolescents," *American Journal of Orthopsychiatry* 51 (1981): 439-453.

12. J. R. Lion, W. Snyder, and G. L. Merrill, "Underreporting of Assaults on Staff in State Hospitals," *Hospital and Community Psychiatry* 32 (1981): 497-498.

13. B. Ekblom, *Acts of Violence by Patients in Mental Hospitals* (Stockholm: Scandanavian University Press, 1970).

14. M. G. Kalogerakis, "The Assaultive Psychiatric Patient," *Psychiatric Quarterly* 45 (1971): 372-381.

15. G. W. Albee, "Patterns of Aggression in Psychopathology," *Journal of Consulting Psychology* 14 (1950): 465-468.

16. R. C. Evenson et al., "Disturbing Behavior: A Study of Incident Reports," *Psychiatric Quarterly* 48 (1974): 266-275.

17. E. Fottrell, "A Study of Violent Behavior Among Patients in Psychiatric Hospitals," *British Journal of Psychiatry* 136 (1980): 216-221.

18. D. Q. Hagen, J. Mikolajczak, and R. Wright, "Aggression in Psychiatric Patients," *Comprehensive Psychiatry* 13 (1972): 481-487.

19. M. Benezech, M. Bourgeois, and J. Yesavage, "Violence and the Mentally Ill: A Study of 547 Patients in a French Hospital for the Criminally Insane," *Journal of Nervous and Mental Disease* 168 (1980): 698-700.

20. K. Tardiff and A. Sweillam, "Assault, Suicide and Mental Illness," *Archives of General Psychiatry* 37 (1980): 164-169.

21. K. Tardiff, "Characteristics of Assaultive Patients in Private Hospitals," *American Journal of Psychiatry*, in press.

22. T. J. Craig, "An Epidemiologic Study of Problems Associated with Violence Among Psychiatric Inpatients," *American Journal of Psychiatry* 139 (1982): 1262-1266.

23. K. Tardiff and A. Sweillam, "The Occurrence of Assaultive Behavior Among Chronic Psychiatric Inpatients," *American Journal of Psychiatry* 139 (1982): 212-215.

24. K. Tardiff and K. Deane, "The Psychological and Physical Status of Chronic Psychiatric Inpatients," *Comprehensive Psychiatry* 21 (1980): 91-97.

25. K. Tardiff, "Emergency Control Measures for Psychiatric Inpatients," *Journal of Nervous and Mental Disease* 169 (1981): 614-618.

26. K. Tardiff, "A Survey of Drugs Used in the Management of Assaultive Inpatients," *Bulletin of the American Academy of Psychiatry and Law* 11 (1983): 215-222.

27. American Medical Association Department of Drugs, *AMA Drug Evaluations,* 4th ed. (Chicago: American Medical Association, 1980).

28. T. M. Itil, "Convulsive and Anticonvulsive Properties of Neuropsychopharmaca in Epilepsy," in *Modern Problems in Pharmacopsychiatry,* ed. E. Niedermeyer (Basel: Karger, 1970).

29. K. Tardiff, "Assault in Hospitals and Placement in the Community," *Bulletin of the American Academy of Psychiatry and Law* 9 (1981): 33-39.

30. S. E. Bruening, "An Applied Dose-response Curve of Thioridazine with the Mentally Retarded: Aggressive, Self-stimulatory, Intellectual and Workshop Behaviors—a Preliminary Report," *Psychopharmacology Reports* 18 (1982): 57-59.

31. R. T. Rada, "The Violent Patient: Rapid Assessment and Management," *Psychosomatics* 22 (1981): 101-109.

32. J. R. Lion and S. A. Pasternak, "Countertransference Reactions to Violent Patients," *American Journal of Psychiatry* 130 (1973): 207-210.

33. J. R. Lion, *"Evaluation and Management of the Violent Patient* (Springfield, Ill.: Charles C Thomas, 1972).

34. K. Tardiff, *The Psychiatric Uses of Seclusion and Restraint* (Washington, D.C.: The American Psychiatric Press, 1984).

35. P. T. Donlon, J. Hopkin, and J. P. Tupin, "Overview: Efficacy and Safety of the Rapid Neuroleptization Method with Injectable Haloperidol," *American Journal of Psychiatry* 136 (1979): 273-278.

36. J. P. Tupin, "Management of Violent Patients," in *A Manual of Psychiatric Therapeutics,* ed. R. Shader (Boston: Little, Brown and Company, 1979).

37. D. J. Madden, "Psychotherapy and Other Traditional Approaches to Managing Violence," in *Clinical Treatment and Management of the Violent Person*, ed. L. Roth (Rockville, Md.: Center for Studies of Crime and Delinquency, National Institutes of Mental Health, 1984).

38. *Youngberg v. Romeo*, 102 S. Ct. 2452 (1982).

39. *Mills v. Rogers*, 102 S. Ct. 2442 (1982).

Chapter 4

Violence: The Emergency Room Patient

Keith A. Wood, Ph.D., and Radwan Khuri, M.D.

INTRODUCTION

A 35-year-old hospital security guard was killed by multiple stab wounds on a walkway between two sections of the medical complex. He was last seen alive when he was called to the emergency room by a receptionist who complained about a demanding patient. The security guard told the patient to calm down and to leave the emergency room immediately after he had been treated. The security guard was subsequently found lying in a pool of blood with multiple stab wounds in his back. The murderer remains at large.

Rates of violent acts are continually increasing, in spite of efforts to reduce or even control such incidents. It has become a major national public health issue, enhancing our fears and taxing our defenses. Both criminal justice and mental health experts have been frustrated in their efforts to predict or rehabilitate individuals who use violence. Such failures in dealing effectively with this social problem have led to a redirection of energies from controlling the actual violence to dealing with its victims.[1,2] While helping a victim of violence is important, helping a potential victim avoid violence is more important. This chapter focuses on both aspects of violence in hospital emergency rooms.

Although violence can occur anywhere, it is more likely to occur in certain settings. It has been well documented that assaultive acts are quite frequent in prisons and ghetto populations, perhaps as a result of the increased presence and recordings of legal authorities in such areas, but violence, although less publicized, frequently occurs in hospital emergency rooms.

Even though there are few studies on violence in health care settings, recent reports point to the emergency room as one area in the hospital where violence is most likely to occur. One study found that 40 percent of emergency room physicians carry handguns into emergency departments for self-protection.[3] In many ways, emergency rooms are accessible arenas for violence. They are unlocked seven days a week, 24 hours a day. They are easily found, and many are in the middle of crime-based neighborhoods. They are full of accessible drugs, women, and hostages. They are typically lacking in security. Emergency room staff members are usually untrained to handle violent situations and weapons easily can be used against them.[4]

Emergency rooms typically are full of tension.[5] Stressed patients, family members, friends, and staff too often interact in a disruptive manner. Emergency room patients are often recipients of violent actions that they have instigated and are eager to continue, frequently against the nearest available person. In an emergency room, some patients, family members, and friends are intoxicated or are withdrawing from a substance and are in a hyperagitated state. Others may have poor impulse control secondary to a psychiatric illness. Still other emergency room violence is initiated by staff members. Those giving the shots, asking the questions, or performing the physicals can induce a disruptive interaction by not considering the patient or by being upset about something else.

The pressure of the hospital emergency room combined with the increased random violence in our society has resulted in multiple aggressive outbursts in emergency rooms throughout this country. Unfortunately, the majority of such acts are not recorded.[6] Emergency personnel typically avoid reporting such incidents because of the additional paper work required, the common occurrence of such aggression, the suggestion that there exists a failure on their part, and the fear of an investigation of their means of self-defense. This under-reporting of assaultive acts has limited our study of factors associated with hospital violence, which some estimate to be five times that reported.[6,7] Despite the limited reporting, we now know some specific factors associated with emergency room violence. This chapter focuses on those factors and various aspects of assessing, controlling, and preventing such incidents.

THEORETICAL MODELS OF AGGRESSION

"I don't know why she attacked the emergency room physician. She has always seemed a bit angry and acted out quite a bit as a child. She caused her family a great deal of trouble. She is a lot like her uncle who is in prison for attempted murder. You know, she's been going through some rough times and has really had to fight to survive. For all I know, she could have been full of drugs. When things build up, who knows what can happen."

Emergency room violence can be dealt with before or after it happens.[8] Unfortunately, most emergency room personnel react to, rather than prevent, violence. Typically, a security guard is called to handle the problem patient. Training in how to "handle the aggressive person's outburst," in holds, take-downs, and restraining procedures is important, but an emphasis on prevention and de-escalation of a potentially violent patient would be preferable.[9] This proactive approach places more responsibility for occur-rences of emergency room violence on the staff's omission or commission of some act, and not solely on the patient or visitor.[9] Preventing violence requires some conceptual understanding of human aggression and some of the major theories by which it is explained.

One theory is that man is instinctually aggressive.[10] Theorists suggest that humans have evolved into their present dominant state by being aggressors who took care of their needs first. To submit was to become extinct; to fight was to survive. This survival characteristic became part of human nature and was passed on genetically. Now, when humans are threatened, their natural response is to become aggressive. In a strange environment like the emergency room, with instruments, staff members, and illnesses threatening to take control, patients and visitors should be expected to react in some aggressive form. A good emergency room plan would aid in the release of aggression in nonviolent forms.

Others view aggression as an innate source of energy.[11] Humans, they feel, are naturally aggressive, even when they are not threatened, and need to release this pent-up energy. For most people, this release occurs in socially acceptable forms in such arenas as business, athletics, politics, or the medical profession. When circumstances limit such releases, aggression is likely to show itself in violent forms. With the restricted avenues for expression in an emergency room, with its strange environment, language, and population, the potential for aggressive outbursts is great.

Still others suggest violence is learned through imitation or experience.[12] Recent studies showing that television violence increases the likelihood of childhood aggression support such theorists.[13] When children observe that individuals who scream, threaten, or fight tend to be more successful, this increases the likelihood that these children will learn to scream, threaten, or fight to get what they want. Aggression, even violence, is rewarded. Some individuals may even look for places or situations in which to enjoy being violent. Unfortunately, many of them end up in emergency rooms secondary to someone else's aggression, still ready to show off their macho images again.

A popular theory asserts that aggression is a result of frustration. This frustration-aggression hypothesis holds that when frustration reaches certain levels, the only release available is aggression.[14] Different individuals find different things frustrating and have different tolerances for frustrations; but each person has a breaking point. Perhaps the frustrations felt prior to admission to the emergency room combine with those experienced while in the emergency room to increase the probability of aggressive behavior. There is quite a bit of literature suggesting that stress does increase the likelihood of aggressive acts.

Some social theorists suggest that aggression is more a territorial issue than an internal event.[15] They posit that each person has various layers of personal space reserved for different degrees of closeness. An outer layer may be for friends, a middle layer for family members, and an inner layer for themselves. When the boundaries of these layers of space are violated, the likelihood of violence increases. Research on personal space also suggests that some individuals react with irritation and hostility when that space is violated.[16] Such individuals would have difficulty with a crowded, hurried emergency room where patients are stretcher to stretcher, and emergency room personnel are sticking, grabbing, touching, and holding without much permission. In these situations, it is a wonder that there aren't even more violent outbursts.

No one theory can completely explain all violence, but theories do help us to be more aware and knowledgeable. In each theory noted, there are traceable influences on human aggression that are directly applicable to the emergency room setting. In each theory, there are environmental factors that could be used to increase or decrease the likelihood of violent behavior or feelings of aggression. Though not fact, each theory gives us some clues as to factors causing or increasing the likelihood of emergency room violence.

FACTORS INCREASING POTENTIAL VIOLENCE

He was brought to the emergency room by the police. His eyes seemed to be bulging out of his head, his mouth was open wide, and he was grunting strange animal-like sounds. Initial attempts to get him to say something intelligible failed. He kept pointing to his stomach and appeared to be choking. Through his hand signals it was determined that he thought someone had put a snake into his stomach that was eating his insides out. He also felt some of the emergency room personnel were involved in the act. When he did begin to speak, he threatened some of them with violence if the snake wasn't stopped. One attendant laughed at the ridiculousness of the patient's delusion. Laboratory tests were positive for various chemicals and verified an organic delusional disorder. While under the influence of these drugs the patient was quite violent. When he was clear of them he was quite friendly.

Some specific factors that increase the likelihood of violence too often are ignored. Various forms of alcohol and drug dependence; systemic, neurological, and organic disorders; functional psychoses and nonpsychotic presentations all increase the risk of disruptive violence in the emergency room.

Patients with alcohol and drug dependence enter emergency rooms in various acute states of intoxication and withdrawal.[17,18] The disinhibiting affect of alcohol or sedative-hypnotic intoxication, the bad trips from hallucinogen and PCP abuse, the overstimulation of the central nervous system by amphetamine or cocaine intoxication, and alcohol or sedative-hypnotic withdrawal all can lead to delirious violent behavior. Paranoid reactions associated with substance abuse, such as alcohol hallucinosis and amphetamine psychosis, may induce physical reactions to imagined dangers. Toxic levels of pharmacological agents can lead to confusion, agitation, and fighting. Anticholinergic and sympathomimetic agents, anticonvulsant and analgesic drugs, digitalis, cimetidine, steroids, levodopa, heavy metals, and other chemical agents have been associated with violent reactions.[18,19] Elderly patients especially are prone to such reactions, even to therapeutic doses. In addition, the elderly are more likely to have paradoxical rage reactions to benzodiazepine or barbiturates.[20]

Mental changes leading to aggressive behavior are a common manifestation of many systemic disorders.[18,19] Electrolyte imbalance, nutritional and vitamin deficiencies, anemia, hypoglycemia, and diabetes are metabolic disturbances that need to be ruled out as causes for aggressive outbursts. Endocrinopathies commonly involving the thyroid and adrenal functions; vital organ failures, such as those resulting in uremia, hepatic encephalopathy, pulmonary insufficiency, or diminished cardiac output; and connective tissue disorders may result in organic brain syndromes that increase the potential for violence. Many such disorders actually may be disguised by a concurrent psychiatric disorder, and thus overlooked.

Neurological disorders, such as head trauma, central nervous system infections, epilepsy in its ictal and postictal psychotic forms, degenerative dementias, and cerebrovascular disease also may be manifested by those exhibiting violent episodes.[18,19] Hypertensive encephalopathy, meningitis, temporal lobe epilepsy, and intracranial hemorrhage or infarct should be investigated quickly as possible causes of sudden changes in behavior.

It is important to emphasize that the presence of a biological insult often serves to intensify borderline paranoid and violent personality features, and does not rule out the role of psychosocial stressors in triggering the violent behavior.

Functional psychoses are a very common precipitant of violence in emergency room settings.[17,18,19] Affective, schizophrenic, and other atypical psychoses are most commonly involved. The euphoric mood of a manic patient may be absent or may give way quickly to a highly irritable and belligerent attitude. Such patients are very easy to provoke and become most violent when their own course of thinking or conversation is interrupted or counteracted.[21] The presence of paranoid delusions in such patients increases the likelihood of physical disruption. Impulse control and frustration tolerance become almost negligible during a full-blown manic episode.

Among schizophrenic patients, violence may result from a wider array of causes. A schizophrenic's disintegrated personality structure increases the likelihood of both provoked and unprovoked violent urges.[22] Command auditory hallucinations may entice patients to commit acts they would not otherwise perform. Delusions of being persecuted often result in action against the "persecutor." During an evaluation session, the exploratory attitude of the examiner may threaten to expose internal chaotic feelings and intensify the patient's retaliatory anger. Those with catatonic forms of schizophrenia may go through phases of excitement where extreme psycho-motor hyperactivity results in purposeless, destructive violence.

In addition to manic and schizophrenic patients, those who develop other types of vaguely classified paranoid psychoses and reactive psychoses are also prone to violence by virtue of their detachment from reality, their loss of impulse control, and their paranoid misinterpretations of their environ-ments.[23] Even though most patients with depression lack the initiative and energy to commit violent acts, some of them have been reported to resort to violent action as a last manifestation of their hopelessness and despair. Some hysterical reactions are in psychotic proportions and are acted out in a potentially dangerous fashion.[22] Functional psychoses, combined with certain psychosocial stressors or the patient's cultural background and personality, significantly modulate the potential for violence.

Compared to psychotic violence, nonpsychotic violence is more easily understood as a logical interaction between the patient's functioning and nonfunctioning coping mechanisms and situational stressors.[24] Emergency room stressors are usually secondary to the patients' health problems or may develop as a result of their interactions with the emergency room setting. Emergency patients presenting with physical illness or trauma commonly experience a number of dysphoric feelings, including a fear of the conse-quences of their illnesses, guilt over their perceived roles in the disease process, fear of rejection by their relatives, fear and guilt over being incapacitated and unable to fulfill their regular duties, and frustration at the loss of control their illnesses cause them.[25] Many patients are prone to transform these experiences into anger, which is intensified by the unfamiliar, highly charged emergency room atmosphere. A prolonged waiting period may be all patients need to pour their anger out on those around them. During the treatment phase, the patient is subjected to intensive interventions, ranging from painful injections to gastric lavage to involuntary restraints. Experiencing such major, sudden invasion of privacy and territoriality combined with less personal supportive care than expected in such settings can lead to escalating anger and a breakdown of impulse control. In addition, some patients present with nonphysical adjustment problems and already show evidence of coping difficulties. In the emergency room, they are more susceptible to foster disruptive feelings, project them on others, and act out in a violent manner.

Manipulative patients who use physical or psychiatric complaints to gain access to drugs, food, or lodging frequently will break out in violence when their motives are discovered or their desires denied.[26] The interaction of a large number of psychological and situational factors in emergency rooms can even trigger aggressive behavior in otherwise mentally stable individuals. In the strange, impersonal atmosphere of emergency rooms, family members and friends, in addition to patients, experience frustrations that could erupt in violence.

Whether the patient's violence in the emergency room results from a psychotic process or from a psychosocially understandable sequence of events, personality patterns significantly contribute to its likelihood.[26,27] Patients coming from disadvantaged socioeconomic groups tend to be less tolerant of frustration and more prone to acting out. Personality styles that include such features as suspiciousness, touchiness, aggressiveness, demandingness, lack of moral values, poor impulse control, and a tendency toward explosive anger are usually overrepresented in a group of violent patients. Diagnostically, patients with antisocial personalities have a long history of violent behavior, emotional callousness, impulsivity, and manipulativeness. Patients with borderline personalities lack the adequate ego strength to control their intense emotional drives and repeatedly exhibit anger outbursts. Those with paranoid personalities are constantly on guard anticipating external danger; their thresholds of violence are usually lower than those of others. Patients with an explosive personality seem prone to suddenly escalating episodes of anger and violence separated by normal periods. Many types of immature personality styles exhibit a recurrent pattern of temper tantrums in the face of stress.

SIGNALS OF IMPENDING VIOLENCE

A twenty-eight-year-old male was brought to the emergency room by the police after reporting that there were people trying to kill him. During the interview, it was discovered that he was actually an undercover agent, but he also had a problem with drug abuse. When his complaints were ignored and his requests for morphine and hospitalization were denied, he became quite upset. His demands increased with the time he spent in the emergency room. He eventually agreed to be released into his wife's custody, but was obviously displeased by the decision. Feeling uncomfortable with this patient, one emergency room physician released him from the restraints while the patient waited for his wife to arrive. He began pacing and cursing. Within a few minutes he was fighting someone who was walking in for treatment.

Preventing violent outbursts should be a major goal in emergency rooms. To accomplish this, the staff must be aware of factors influencing their likelihood. A general understanding of the psychotic and nonpsychotic causes is a first step in that direction. A second step involves sensitivity to the large number of clues derived from the patient's behavior and psychosocial history that can alert the observer to the possibility of impending violence.

Demographic Information

The patient's age, sex, race, and family situation can be relevant to potential violence.[28,30] Young males, particularly those between the ages of fifteen and thirty, tend to be the most violent subgroup, both within and outside the hospital environment.[29] Blacks, who have more reported criminal activity in the general population, are not significantly more violent in hospital settings.[29]

Patients with no social restraints, such as spouses or children, tend to be more violent than those that do, but for patients that do have family members, those family members can also provide specific targets for violence.[24]

Immediate Situation

In assessing potential for violence, it is important to determine the patient's living arrangements immediately preceding and following admission.[9] What is the home environment like? Is it supportive? Is it antagonistic? Are family members prone toward aggression? Is the patient taking medications? Are they available? What are the side effects? What is the patient's general response? Does the patient have any available means of assault? Does the patient possess a knife or gun? Are there ink pens or pencils available to stab with? Has the patient identified someone as a target for violence? Is that person accessible to the patient?

Recent History

Recent suggestive actions may be the only signals of aggressive potential. Cleaning or examining one's gun for no obvious purpose, purchasing ammunition, or driving 90 miles an hour after a quarrel are suspicious behaviors. A woman who complains of uneasiness bordering on panic each time she walks in the kitchen may reveal a frightening impulse to jab a knife into her child. A housewife who reports having thrown out all the pills in the medicine cabinet may have done so to prevent hurting herself. A father who gets frustrated with his baby's crying may burst out of the house before harming his child. A wife may report that her husband has nearly strangled her on two or three recent occasions, or threatened her with a knife when he was drunk. A patient who desperately has been seeking help by calling relatives, visiting a minister, and shopping for doctors may be attempting to keep threatening internal urges under control. Such examples illustrate how recent behavior may be a clue to potential violence in emergency room settings.[24]

Family Conflicts

Approximately 25 percent of all reported homicides are between family members, and half of those are between husbands and wives. In one study, 41 percent of women killed were murdered by their husbands, and 11 percent of murdered men were killed by their wives.[26] Such family violence may take place in the highly charged atmosphere of an emergency room; thus, statements regarding family conflicts should never be taken lightly. Moreover, circumstances surrounding a significant relative of the patient may trigger a violent response in the emergency room. Discovery of infidelity, insults, or loss through separation or death of a close relative are likely to stimulate the vulnerable patient to become violent in this setting.

Past and Early History

The best predictor of future violence is the history of violence.[24] A history of homicides or assaultive acts with the infliction of physical injury suggests a chronically low threshold for anxiety, frustration, and anger with accompanying difficulty controlling aggressive impulses. Patients who verbally threaten violence are as likely to be violent as those with a history of violence.[24]

Certain factors in childhood and adolescence appear to be associated with an increased risk of developing a lifelong pattern of violent behavior.[24] Primary among these is severe emotional deprivation or overt rejection in childhood. These commonly occur in chaotic family environments. Multiple foster home experiences, parental seduction ranging from subtle forms to frank incest, and exposure to brutality and extreme violence in early development as a witness or a subject increase the probability of future aggressiveness. Childhood behaviors, such as fire setting, cruelty to animals, uncontrollable temper tantrums, school truancy, excessive fighting, and late bedwetting are early signs of an aggressive coping style.

Mental Status Examination

To the alert clinician, the most obvious signs of impending aggression tend to be reflected in the patient's disrupted mental attitude.[17] The confusion, irrational thinking, and excitement of delirium lowers a patient's impulse control, which could easily lead to aggression. Verbal and nonverbal clues may precede the onset of violence. Usually, the mere attitude of careful listening will alert the staff to what may be upcoming. Patients who express anger, frustration, or violent intentions, boast of prior violence, or relate fears of losing control over impulses should be taken at their word. Nonverbal clues indicating potential for violence include nervous pacing, muscle tensing, increased rates of breathing, twitching of the eyelids, and threatening gestures.[23] The agitation of mania or paranoid thoughts of schizophrenia also may lead to violent episodes. Patients who display many tatoos on their bodies or present to the emergency room with gangs commonly exhibit lower thresholds to violent action.[4] The gut feelings of the examiner are best heeded. Quite often, those feelings lead the health care professional to an accurate prediction of the patient's behavior, even in the absence of more objective clues.[17]

MANAGEMENT OF IMPENDING VIOLENCE

While sitting at her desk, the emergency room physician turned around to see a former patient entering her office. She immediately noticed that he had a gun pointed directly toward her. She felt trapped, with no place to go. Her skin became hot, her heart beat rapidly, and she almost panicked. As slowly and as calmly as she could under the circumstances, she said, "I see you have a gun."

Once a chance of violence has been recognized, the goals of keeping peace and preventing harm obligate the staff to take definitive steps toward avoiding confrontation.[5] This is especially difficult when patients directly threaten those in charge of their care. Above all, the staff should not act on their own natural inclinations to match the threats. Instead, it is crucial to understand the patients' viewpoints and attempt to help them master their frustrations and manipulate their environments so that they feel more secure.[21] Since violent patients actually feel trapped, afraid, frustrated, insecure, and vulnerable, the last thing they need is for anyone to exacerbate those anxieties by projecting a macho or threatening image. To help de-escalate the potential for violence, it is important to assume the role of the patient's advocate.[31] It is helpful initially to engage the patient in a calm, self-assured voice and ask, "How can I help you?" This offer alone often relieves much of the frustration and anxiety and makes the patient feel more secure because someone cares. A further offer of food or drink also serves to lessen the patient's uncomfortable state, since it gives or projects an interest in his or her welfare. It is also important to show no anxiety or fear. Once a patient relaxes to some degree, you can establish the potential for violence by asking, "What are your feelings about becoming violent?" Or, "What fears have you had about losing control and hurting someone?" This allows the patient to deal with any violent impulses in a more socially acceptable manner through verbalization.

In addition to presenting a calm, caring attitude, you should put patients at ease physically.[17] The following steps are helpful in accomplishing this. First, try to interview patients alone; this helps them feel less vulnerable and minimizes the possibility of threatening actions by other emergency staff members or patients. However, interviewers should never place themselves in situations of probable harm. Patients should always be asked if they possess any weapons. In cases where patients are extremely agitated or paranoid, they should be interviewed either in a large room or in a hall. Second, choose an area for the interview that is as private as possible and away from the confusion of the emergency room and other disturbed or provocative patients. Third, don't leave the patients alone in a room. Disturbed patients may interpret this as rejection, and it provides an opportunity for them to hurt themselves. If the interviewer must leave, another staff member or security guard should remain near the door or in the room so the patient at least feels someone's presence. Fourth, never approach potentially violent patients rapidly or get too close to them. It is always wise to stay at least an arm's length away and choose a position in which easy escape is possible if there are aggressive outbursts.

If patients appear quite angry, it is helpful to acknowledge their anger.[4] This communicates an understanding of the strong emotions they are experiencing. The technique of making an observation frequently defuses tense situations. When you don't know what else to do, make an observation.[5] Say something like, "I see you are very upset. Would you mind telling me what is causing these feelings?"

It is also quite helpful to encourage the patient to help solve the problem.[4] This technique is also quite useful with family members or friends. In crisis situations, people tend to panic and to blame, especially to point a finger at those in authority. They often interfere with the resolution. By engaging the patient, the family, or friends in handling the conflict, you can defuse much of their interference.

With patients who are severely agitated and may not be in touch with reality, first evaluate the situation and determine the degree of danger: Where are you? Where is the patient? How agitated is the patient? Next, acknowledge the patient's predicament and agitation, offer help, and set limits. Remember, such individuals have poor impulse control and need someone in a role of authority to help them establish some confidence. Try saying patiently, firmly, and respectfully, "Please sit down." Or, "I want to help you, but you must sit down and then I'll be right with you." That displays the control the patient somehow knows is needed. The next step is to explore: "I see that you are upset and agitated. Tell me, do you feel dangerous to yourself or others?" If the answer is that they do feel dangerous to someone, find out to whom. Have the patient specify with whom they are upset. Then ask, "Would you like to be restrained?" Setting limits is important for such patients.

Some patients will not respond to the verbal and physical comforts outlined above. Instead, they will remain anxious and disorganized. These patients require assurance that violent behavior is unacceptable. Sometimes, a final, firm, verbal warning suffices. If this appears ineffective, a visual warning may work.[31] Assemble a group of four or five security personnel and advise them of the patient's problems and of their own specific roles. They should remain within calling distance at all times in case trouble occurs or verbal warnings fail to quiet a patient. It helps to use a code word, such as "Dr. Armstrong," to avoid further agitating the patient when calling security. Upon summons by the staff member, the security officers should appear before the patient so their presence can be seen and felt. This "show of force" indicates that any display of violence will not be tolerated, and often helps disorganized patients to gain control of their thoughts and behavior. If these techniques fail, medication may be needed.

The following is a list of recommendations regarding the common mistakes that may be committed while dealing with a potentially violent situation:

1. Don't deny the possibility of violence when you start recognizing early clues to escalating agitation in the patient's behavior. Also, don't underestimate information given by others regarding such clues.
2. Don't isolate yourself with a potentially violent patient unless you have made sure that enough security measures have been taken to prevent or limit a harmful violent outburst.
3. Avoid certain behaviors that may be interpreted as aggressive, such as moving too close to the patient, touching, staring directly into their eyes, speaking loudly, displaying facial expressions or body movements of a threatening nature, or allowing several staff members to interact simultaneously with the patient.
4. Don't make promises you can't keep.
5. Don't allow your feelings of fear, anger, or hostility to interfere with your self-control and professional understanding of the patient's circumstances. Don't argue, give orders, or disagree when not necessary.

In summary, to deal effectively with the potentially violent patient, it is necessary to understand and accurately assess the patient's mental state, to use therapeutic techniques to help de-escalate the tension, to maintain self-control of personal emotions that may counteract therapeutic efforts, and to stay aware of the security factors relevant to this potentially explosive situation.

HANDLING THE OCCURRENCE OF VIOLENCE

An attractive thirty-two-year-old female ran to a hospital's emergency room and said that she had been raped by two men—her husband and a neighbor. During an investigation by the police, she claimed some of the emergency room staff also raped her. The staff, fearing this was a sign of a serious mental illness, had her restrained for assessment by the psychiatric service. She initially refused to talk to the doctors. When eventually she did speak, it was of her helpless state and how hard it was for her to be held against her will. She cried when talking about her circumstances, which seemed to be caused by her passivity. While she was being escorted to the restroom, she broke away from a police officer. She ran through the emergency room, with two policemen, one policewoman, a security guard, and various staff members chasing her. When they caught her, they immediately tried to wrestle her down. Two got hurt in the process. The police reacted by becoming more aggressive, carrying the patient to a stretcher and chaining her arms and legs to it.

Once violent behavior occurs, immediate action is called upon to subdue patients and assure their protection.[5] First, the area should be cleared immediately. A team of five people is needed to control the patient, one to hold each limb and one to apply physical restraints. While the restraints are being placed on, it is advisable to explain to the patient what is being done and why. Two restraints are usually the minimum required to keep the patient on a stretcher. As soon as control is obtained, the patient should be checked for weapons, sharp instruments, or drugs. Throughout this process, it is important to continually reassure patients about the staff's concern for their safety and to help them tone down their agitation with various verbal suggestions.

Ideally, an adequate diagnostic evaluation attending to etiological factors should be made before medicating the patient. However, if the patient remains agitated in spite of the physical restraints and verbal interventions, symptomatic treatment with a psychotropic agent may prove necessary.[32] The safest sedating agent to use when diagnostic clues are still lacking is haloperidol, an antipsychotic phenothiazine agent that has effective sedating properties and poses no risk of cardiorespiratory depression.[33] Haloperidol's antipsychotic properties are also highly useful in resolving psychotic symptoms that commonly underlie violent behavior in the emergency room. The dosage should be five to ten mg intramuscularly and may be repeated after an hour if clinically indicated. Other antipsychotic agents with a low risk of autonomic side effects may also be used.[33] Antipsychotic sedation may pose a risk of decreased seizure threshold with seizure-prone patients, including those with bona fide epilepsy, and those in alcohol or sedative-hypnotic withdrawal or in stimulant intoxication. The use of sedative hypnotics and anxiolytic agents, such as barbiturates or benzodiazepines, should be avoided when the patient's diagnosis is unclear; they may cause severe central nervous system depression leading to grave consequences in a subgroup of delirious patients.

When the underlying diagnosis is clear, treatment strategies then can be applied in a more appropriate fashion. Chemotherapy and crisis intervention are the two main lines of intervention in such circumstances. Psychotic patients are commonly beyond the reach of mere psychotherapeutic efforts, and chemotherapy often proves essential to their treatment. Benzodiazepines are useful in the treatment of alcohol or sedative-hypnotic withdrawal and amphetamine or other central nervous system stimulant intoxication states.[32]

In addition, reports have warned that hallucinogen-induced psychoses may get worse with antipsychotic treatment and that the use of benzodiazepines should be the first choice of treatment. Finally, anticholinergic toxic psychoses respond favorably to benzodiazepines, whereas the anticholinergic properties of antipsychotic agents make the use of the latter group contraindicated.

Antipsychotic agents, such as haloperidol, chlorpromazine, fluphenazine, thiothixene, thioridazine, and others, are very effective in the treatment of psychotic behavior associated with functional and organic psychoses other than those mentioned above. High-potency, low-dosage compounds have minimal autonomic side effects, but a high incidence of extrapyramidal reactions. They are safer to use with elderly or cardiovascular patients. The high-dosage, low-potency group of antipsychotic agents is preferable for use with young, healthy patients. With elderly patients, who have a decreased ability to metabolize and excrete various pharmacological agents, dosages should be reduced. Because of their addictive potential, sedative hypnotics in the emergency room should only be used in the clinical situations described earlier. Their frequent use in a general emergency room invites an increasing number of substance abusers seeking treatment with such agents.[18]

When the patient's violence is not caused by a psychotic process, crisis intervention is the treatment of choice, whether or not chemical restraints are used. A thorough evaluation of the psychosocial factors that activated the violent behavior should be undertaken. Crisis intervention with a supportive thrust should be initiated to address the specific conflicts with which the patient is struggling. A problem-solving approach or analytical techniques may be indicated as part of the short-term therapeutic intervention. Manipulative patients often require a limit-setting, confrontational approach, and behavioral methods may be needed to shape their behavior into more adaptive modes.

Where indicated, family therapy in the emergency room may help address interpersonal family conflicts that could have contributed to the violent behavior. An active, confrontational problem-solving approach is quite useful in this treatment context.

If emergency interventions are ineffective or insufficient, serious consideration should be given to hospitalizing the patient. The patient's violent behavior may require involuntary commitment procedures if the condition continues to threaten the patient's safety or that of others.[19] Where hospitalization is not indicated, an adequate outpatient treatment plan should be initiated as appropriate to the patient's medical and psychiatric status.

COMMITMENT ISSUES

A young male was brought to the emergency room by the police after getting into a fight with his brother for no obvious reason. His mother called complaining of her son's increased hostility and uncontrollable behavior. In the emergency room, he explained how his family was against him because he was not studying in college as his two brothers did. He appeared very confident in his ability to handle his situation and felt no need for psychiatric help. He denied any homicidal or suicidal thoughts or plans, but he did have a history of aggressive threats and acts. The psychiatric consultant recommended releasing him from the emergency room and referring him for outpatient treatment, even though he was still in an agitated state. His family refused to accept him at their home, which only made him more upset. He went to an aunt's house to spend the night. The following morning he became quite agitated with this aunt; they argued and fought. In a state of rage, he got a knife and stabbed her 43 times, all over her body. She was found dead in a pool of blood. The family now plans to sue the hospital.

Assessing the competence of emergency room patients threatening or committing violent acts is an increasingly important legal issue.[34] When the violent behavior occurs in the context of a psychotic mental state, the emergency room physician (and in some states, the clinical psychologist) has the power and the duty to initiate commitment procedures. This allows the physician to initiate involuntary treatment and/or hospitalization in order to protect the patient and the immediate environment and to treat the underlying mental disorder that is assumed to be one cause of the violence.[19,27] The basic assumption underlying the procedure of emergency commitment is that the patient cannot be held legally responsible for imminent or actual violence when that person is suffering from an altered mental state. On the other hand, if the violent behavior occurs in the absence of a mental disorder of psychotic proportions, the physician in the emergency room must depend on security and police officials to control the violence and initiate the legal steps that would naturally follow any similar incident in any other setting. Thus, the assessment of the mental condition of the violent patient is crucial in determining how far the emergency room physician is allowed to go in intervening and when the case should be turned over to law enforcement officials. The liability of the emergency room staff and of the sponsoring hospital is most obvious when clinicians fail to recognize their duty to commit a psychotically violent patient to involuntary treatment and when further violent behavior later invites legal action against the medical institution and the clinician in question.

Patients have the right to confidentiality, except when their behavior takes on a violent dimension requiring emergency interventions.[4] In dealing with the violent emergency room patient, all attempts should be made to secure as much information as possible about the patient's condition in order to ensure rapid protection for all involved. This is even more important now that legal authorities are increasing their concern for the rights of victims of violence.

Thus, in general, legal difficulties resulting from emergency room violence are determined more often by errors of omission than by errors of commission. Emergency intervention, whether medical or legal, has to be swift and effective.

STAFF REACTIONS TO VIOLENCE

> "It really wasn't as bad as people made it out to be. Patients act out all the time. I should have known better than to touch her when I did. After all, I've been working in the emergency room for a long time and know I was likely to get hurt at least once. Besides, I felt there was something strange about that patient. I guess my mind was on something else. In some ways I feel guilty about this whole incident. You know, if I hadn't done a few things to agitate her, I wouldn't have gotten hurt, and she would have received better care. If it's anybody's fault, it's the hospital's. They overwork us and just are not concerned about our reactions in situations like this. If I could have avoided it, I wouldn't have reported this incident; I knew they wouldn't do anything but give me a hassle. I'll just have to be more careful in the future."

The longer an individual works in an emergency room, the more likely it becomes that that person will be assaulted by a patient.[7] Such assaults generally include being grabbed, hit in the ear and jaw, choked, knocked down, and thrown to the floor. In most cases where staff members have been attacked, the staff members were aware of the patient's potential toward violence.[7]

Being the victim of violence by emergency room patients can result in loss of time from work and the need for various forms of treatment. Some staff members have had only bruised feelings, while others require treatment ranging from first aid to hospitalization. There are reports of emergency room patients actually killing emergency room personnel.

Hospital staff members who have been victims of patient violence generally report minimal reactions. Some feel they would be overwhelmed if they allow themselves to admit their inner feelings about being assaulted. Others indicate that patient violence could prevent them from doing their jobs, was part of their jobs, or was to be expected.

In general, emergency room staff members who are recipients of violence report such short-term emotional reactions as anger, anxiety, helplessness, irritability, feelings of resignation, sadness, depression, shock, apathy, disbelief, self-blame, dependence, fear of returning to the scene of the assaults, fear of others, feeling sorry for the patients who committed the assaults, and feeling that they should have done something to prevent the assault.[7,32] In many cases, such staff members either deny or rationalize the violent act: "I don't even think about it. There's always a good side; I focus on the positive. I don't feel remorse or revenge." In other cases, staff members are more preoccupied with the assaults, experiencing guilt and self-blame. They tend to focus on psychological and somatic reactions to the violent episodes: "This is not the patient's fault. I should have been more careful and restrained the patient more. Perhaps he felt my tenseness and became more anxious and violent." "I wonder if this incident will make me more afraid of all strangers. I hope I don't start a pattern of headaches from the hit. Perhaps I am the type of person an angry person would hit! Maybe I shouldn't work in an emergency room setting." Victims of an assault also have some social reactions which are revealed in changes in relationships with co-workers and difficulty in returning to work. Biophysical reactions, such as startle responses, sleep pattern disturbances, soreness, and headaches are common short-term reactions.

Many of the short-term reactions dissipate in a week or so, but there are also long-term reactions that can last anywhere from a week to a year. On an emotional level, feelings of anger, anxiety, and fear of, and concern for, the patient who committed the assault typically continue past the first week.[7] Some individuals try to deny or rationalize these feelings: "The injury was an accident. The patient was confused, not in his right mind, and thus not totally responsible." Or, "It was my stupidity. I should have called for help sooner." There are also continued biophysiological reactions, such as concern about long-term physical side effects and an increased sense of vulnerability. Concern about the dangerousness of emergency room work and the lack of protection and administrative support also becomes more important. There is a feeling among some emergency room staff personnel that the administration is primarily concerned about patients' rights and does not care about the rights or safety of the staff.

In summary, reactions to emergency room violence can last much longer than the time the staff member is away from work following an incident. In addition, the staff members typically either fail to report violence or attempt to rationalize any reactions to being victims of violence. This complicates efforts to understand staff reactions to violence, which are probably more significant than present published reports reflect.

SECURITY

The injured child's parents arrived at the emergency room. They didn't seem any different than any other concerned relatives of the sick and injured that pass through any hospital's emergency room on any given day. The father, at first, just expressed the fear and concern expected. His child was in pain, very ill, and he felt powerless to do anything himself. He was in a world totally foreign to him. The language was only vaguely recognizable as English, not what he used with his friends. The smell was even different. He was afraid, helpless, a foreigner in his own neighborhood, and very concerned about his daughter. He expressed his concern in the only way he knew, by asking questions. When he did get an answer, he really didn't understand it. He responded by asking more questions and raising his voice. He didn't want to cause a problem; he was trying to cause a solution. He confronted a number of people dressed in white. They didn't intend to antagonize him; they just had their jobs to do and didn't have the time. They weren't assigned to patient relations. "Somebody will be with you in just a minute," he was told. He felt like he was getting the runaround. As his fear increased, so did his imagination. In desperation, he grabbed somebody dressed in a white coat and demanded some attention and some answers.

Security was called for assistance in handling an aggressive subject in the emergency room. The security officer had been in the army, preferred to be a police officer, but for the past year-and-a-half had been in security. Now he had to deal with some "real trouble" and had double-timed it from the lobby down to the emergency room. As he rushed through the door, he knew the problem: one adult male was shoving an orderly around and yelling at the same time. He grabbed the attacker by the shoulder and spun him around, figuring if he could get him into a wrist come-along and bring him down he could cool the whole thing down. It didn't work out that way.

When the visitor felt himself being grabbed and spun from behind, he really didn't know what was going on. He wasn't aware that he

had done anything really bad. "Here's a cop, he's trying to grab my
arms and do a job on me. I have to defend myself." The officer,
because the subject went berserk, was forced to use a baton, which
in turn left the subject with multiple contusions, lacerations, and a
hairline-fractured skull.[8]

Looking at the cold, hard facts, it is obvious that this situation was not
handled well. Security simply took a bad situation and made it worse.
Another option would have been preferable. Recognizing that the parents
were in a very stressful situation, the security guard could have taken them
into an adjoining waiting area and explained the basic procedures that were
being carried out on their child. By using terms to which they could relate,
the security guard could have suggested that there was information the
parents could provide that might help in the treatment strategy for their
child. By making repeated visits to reassure the parents, the guard would
have been able to reduce their anxieties and aid in their eventual reunion with
their child.

Emergency room security personnel frequently encounter people who are
at the height of physical or mental stress. In such situations, sometimes only
seconds are available in which to deal with the situation. The initial
interaction with an upset visitor, patient, or family member is not the time to
learn what to do. An arbitrary decision at this point could be expected to
cause hostility escalation, physical aggression, or worse.

When a situation gets out of hand, the underlying problem is often that
well-intentioned security personnel failed to contain problems they felt were
not their responsibilities.[9] They tried. The problem is that the progression of a
patient, visitor, or family member from slightly upset to physically violent is
very much the responsibility of those who confront them. For any form of de-
escalation to work, the very first step is for staff members to accept the reality
that their conduct mediates the conduct of the agitated person most of the
time.[9] The stance, attitude, affect, and verbalizations of the staff are critical.
What is said or not said, done or not done, shapes, directs, escalates, de-
escalates, encourages, promotes, causes, and allows the behavior of the person
being confronted. Security personnel must recognize that their behaviors are
reflected by the people to whom they relate. If hostilities are to be contained
and defused, that containment is the responsibility of the officer, not the
hostile individual. Security personnel's ability to defuse hostility depends on
how they feel, how they behave, and how much control they have over
themselves. If the security officer is prejudiced, emotionally involved, or
biased, the individual will sense it.

In viewing a violent individual, it is important that security officers
perceive that person as using violence as a coping mechanism.[25] The patient's

fear of loss of control or internal hostile urges makes violence a means of either combating feelings of helplessness or controlling others. These frightening feelings are increased by harmful staff attitudes, such as a defensive denial of the potential for violent or countertransferent feelings that result in overreaction to, or rejection of, patients. Violent behavior depends not only on what is going on inside the patient biologically or intrapsychically, but also on interactions with the people and things in the environment. Ongoing activity, decor, and staff actions, and the patients' location in relationship to others, have a great deal to do with the patients' behavior.

When dealing with patients in the emergency room, it is important to determine whether they have fears about being in the emergency room, frustrations about why they are there, feelings of rejection by family or staff members, or grief reactions. Determining why a patient is or might become angry helps to prevent or reduce the anger.

It is important for security guards to be aware of their own inner feelings and physiological responses to stress in order to manage emergency room violence properly. Remember personal responses and use them as cues leading to appropriate coping mechanisms, rather than as signals for panic. When a patient is verbally expressing distress, encourage exploration and ventilation, but deal with threatening patients with firm, but supportive, limit setting. (Make sure you can back up your limits.) Brief summaries or directive comments designed to help the patient break a crisis down into a series of small problems that can be handled in nonviolent ways are quite useful. Patients generally appreciate appropriate explanations. They also appreciate staff members who only make promises that can be kept.

Security personnel must develop successful responses to agitated people. Training oneself to instantly assess the emotional status of a person involves intensely watching that person. Look for early warning signs, such as excessive adrenalin production, tense muscles, body position, twitching fingers or eyelids, pacing, jerkiness, or withdrawal as you approach.[9] Listen to the person's voice and breathing. Changes in vocal pitch and an increased respiratory rate may suggest reduced oxygen supply to the brain, which results in reduced clarity in thinking. If you suspect a person is armed, watch the hands. Otherwise, attention should be primarily directed at an imaginary spot on the individual's upper chest, while glancing from time to time at the eyes. Avoid concentrated fixation on the person's eyes; staring might easily be interpreted as an attempt to dominate.[31]

Security guards are often called to de-escalate problems that the medical staff could not handle. The methods for managing such situations are similar to those mentioned for emergency room personnel, but are often more intense. Officers should approach the patient calmly, acting helpful. They should speak and stand in a relaxed manner, but always balanced and prepared to move. The pitch and volume of the voice should be consciously lowered. The speech should be clear and slow, with simple words that are immediately understood. The idea is to get the person talking; then listen to what is said and how it is said. Officers can establish positive communications with someone by how they listen, what they say, and how they say it. Often the source of concern can be identified and help can begin immediately. If not, the officer should keep talking and listening, using time to calm things down.

If the situation presents itself, the security guard could try to distract the person from the immediate causes of their agitation.[4,9] It is amazing how many upset individuals are successfully defused by an offer of coffee, food, or an activity that helps keep their minds off the immediately agitating situation. A negative form of distraction is the presence of other staff personnel attempting to interact with the patient at the same time. This should be avoided with a well-publicized procedure that limits the number of interactors as much as possible. It is useful to invite the patient to sit with the officer to explain the situation, if the confrontation occurs in an environment where that is practical. It should be very clear this is an invitation rather than an order. Both parties should sit down at the same time. If the patient stands, then the security guard must stand. Once both are seated, the officer should maintain a calm, low-pitched voice, signaling that the confrontation need not escalate any further. Staying with the individual until some resolution is achieved is important. If the person makes demands or statements that the officer cannot agree with, the officer shouldn't argue. Arguing creates a no-win situation. The patient may not be logical, and if the officer loses the argument, it may weaken his credibility. Perhaps even more dangerous, officers can become so wrapped up in believing they are right that some loss of self-control may occur in an effort to win the argument. Instead, the officer should try to respond to the emotions that the person is showing. If it is anger, the officer should acknowledge the anger and empathize with the patient. By recognizing that such feelings are real, the officer can work with the individual to resolve them. Officers should never make promises that can't be kept or threats that can't be carried out. They should never offer a reward for that which started out as illegal or improper conduct. Keeping control of behavior, body language, feelings, and expressions is important. When one controls oneself, one controls the situation.

Security guards need to prepare themselves to talk calmly to patients. This requires talking oneself into it. Even under the most stressful situations, the human mind has the remarkable capacity to control the most automatic body functions.[9] Whenever stress is experienced, people tend to tense up various muscle systems, and this is usually very obvious to others. Security guards cannot afford to give such messages. To become more aware of their facial muscles, officers need to study their faces in the mirror. Most facial wrinkles map those muscles a person tightens when upset. By tensing and relaxing facial muscles in front of a mirror, guards can study and become more aware of their presentations. They should confront a hostile person with relaxed muscles during the approach and during the situation itself. It is also important to think clearly under stressful situations. The mind can control the body, but this requires concentration from the earliest moments of arrival on the scene. Officers should look the situation over and check their stances, distances, and responses to the person's needs or emotions. Patients should be given options (not orders) that leave their self-respect intact. This may avoid an attack or a rekindling of the hostile behavior.

PHYSICAL DESIGN OF THE EMERGENCY AREA

He came to the emergency room's admission clerk demanding immediate attention. When told he would "have to wait a few minutes," he became quite upset and stormed from the area. Somewhat relieved, the clerk returned to her normal activities. Five minutes later she heard a scuffle and saw the same man running from the medicine area to the exit. About a minute later, three security guards arrived.

This patient had gone into the medicine area, demanded some medication, became furious when refused, stabbed the physician in the shoulder, knocked down a nurse, and ran out of the emergency room. It happened quickly, and no one was prepared for such an incident.

The design of the emergency department may increase or decrease the potential for violence, help prepare staff for a violent outburst, and help control a violent patient.[35] The patient's environment is an important aspect in determining the likelihood of violent behavior. Unfortunately, few architects have ever been in an emergency room, and even fewer have ever worked in one, so most emergency rooms are based on space and pipe needs instead of patient and security needs. Even so, some simple adjustments can improve almost any emergency room's security.[35]

Installing convex mirrors that permit personnel to see around corners and the entrance and reception area is quite useful. The reception area should have a good view of all other areas, including the front door. There should be no hiding places in the reception area. In some situations, a closed-circuit television would be preferable. Both mirrors and cameras are rather inexpensive, but quite valuable, security devices.

It is beneficial for the emergency room to have a television set in the reception area. It helps waiting patients, friends, and relatives to wile away the time. It also attracts staff members, such as security guards, who might not ordinarily be there during coffee breaks. Seeing security guards can cause some violence-prone individuals to think twice about getting too belligerent.

It is also useful to have a physical barrier of nonbreakable material between the public and the receptionist. This helps to keep people from leaping over the counter and grabbing money or a person as a hostage. Of course, such a barrier could be a bit undesirable, giving a nonviolent patient a negative impression, but in a situation where protection is important, it is a worthwhile security precaution.

An emergency department also requires a multiple alarm system. Panic buttons that can be operated by the receptionist's leg to send a silent alarm either to the central telephone operator, who can call the police or security, or directly to the police station, can be quite helpful. In addition, an automatic telephone calling system, by which one merely takes the phone off the hook to summon help, is a secondary precaution. Occasionally a staff person can call mistakenly and can get a dramatic response from security or law enforcement people, but the security benefits offset such occasional problems.

Automatic telephone dialers are another easy, inexpensive, effective way to get help. It's easier to push one button than to dial a number, even 911. In short, under violence-prone situations, an alarm device that is simple, quick, efficient, effective, and automatic is best.

It is useful for emergency departments to also have radio communication available. Security officers typically carry radio equipment, and it is useful to be able to communicate with them via radio in case other forms of communications are out of order. In every department there needs to be several ways of summoning help.

As discussed in an earlier section of this chapter, people with organic or functional illnesses frequently become violent. Criminals who are brought to the emergency department for a medical or psychiatric check before they are put in jail may become violent. A seclusion room where they can be observed, treated, and kept out of the path of other patients may be beneficial. It is preferable for such a room to have a substantial look, with wire mesh and a heavy door, so a patient inside would think twice before trying to crash out of it. Caution should be used so that there is never an area where patients could find things to hurt themselves or others. The ceiling should not be made of acoustic tile, because the panels could be removed and patients could either gain access to other parts of the hospital or hang themselves. Ceilings should be solid with virtually no openings. The ceiling light should have an unbreakable cover without glass or metal. An examining bed or a vinyl mattress on the floor is the only furniture needed. The room should have an intercom system and a panic button recessed into the wall—something patients can't get to or use as a weapon against others or themselves. When interviewing patients in the seclusion room, it is important for the interviewers to keep their backs to the door and not to the patient. Ideally, the room should have two exits so the interviewers will never be trapped there with the patients and the patients won't feel trapped and become violent. Again, one should never be alone in a closed room with a violent patient.

Another consideration should be the colors used in the emergency department. Some studies have shown that pink has a calming effect, at least for about 20 minutes.

Developing a plan for dealing with a violent patient who gets loose is also important. The staff should know what to do if they are faced with a violent patient or with someone who has a weapon. (Practice sessions should be held.) How do they protect themselves, protect others, and protect hospital property? Staff members should understand what to do during a crisis as clearly as they know what to do when a patient has multiple trauma or experiences a cardiac arrest. Training for hostage survival can be useful in saving the lives of patients, staff, and visitors.[36]

It may be helpful to have a behavioral emergency response team that provides instant staffing when needed. Patients under the influence of PCP or other hallucinogenic drugs are exceptionally violent and strong. Sometimes they seem oblivious to pain and can even snap metal handcuffs. Restraining them requires the muscle power of several trained individuals. A response team should have at least one person for each of the patient's extremities, as well as a team leader who might manage to protect the patient's head so that it isn't bashed on the floor or wall. Most of all, it is important not to try to control a strong person—particularly one under the influence of drugs—with the help of just one or two nurses.

Staff members must think of protecting themselves first, other members of the staff next, and then other patients when dealing with a violent patient. Since staff members know their way out of the emergency department, they can easily head for a closet if bullets start to fly. But patients will not know where to go. Many of them will be in hospital gowns, making escape more difficult. Staff members are never to use themselves as human shields. There are definitely better prevention techniques. A response plan is the best protection.

CONCLUSION

Emergency room violence is not completely random or uncontrollable. To a large extent, its occurrence or nonoccurrence is dependent upon the actions and attitudes of the staff and the physical makeup of the emergency department. Training emergency room employees how to detect signs of potential aggression and de-escalation techniques for patients acting out has not been a priority in most hospitals. Many violent episodes are never documented, and those reported are often vague and confusing due to the lack of attention given to systematic recording methods. Many times there is a lack of sensitivity to the patients' cultural, educational, economic or other differences, and a lack of awareness of staff members' reactions to being victims of patient violence.

Emergency room safety faces new challenges with the general increase in crime, de-institutionalization of psychiatric patients, alternatives to imprisonment, and treatment of drug addicts on an outpatient basis. Specific procedures, specialized training, and structural modifications could become legal requirements in an effort to limit the occurrence and effects of violence in health care settings.

NOTES

1. E. Chelimsky, "Serving Victims: Agency Incentives and Individual's Needs," in *Evaluating Victim Services*, ed. S. E. Salasin (Beverly Hills, California: Sage, 1981).

2. M. Siegal, "Crime and Violence in America: The Victims," *American Psychologist* 38 (1983): 1267-1273.

3. J. Shaw, "Physicians Wonder How to Handle E.R. Violence," *American Medical News*, October 1982, pp. 13-14.

4. E. H. Taliaferro, "The Prepared Emergency," *Emergency Medicine*, May 15, 1983, pp. 27-39.

5. S. Perry, "Effective Management of the Violent," *Emergency Room Reports*, 1983, pp. 31-36.

6. J. R. Lion, G. Bachy Rita, and F. R. Ervin, "Violent Patients in the Emergency Room," *American Journal of Psychiatry* 125 (1969): 1706-1711.

7. M. L. Lanza, "The Reactions of Nursing Staff to Physical Assault by a Patient," *Hospital and Community Psychiatry* 32 (1983): 44-47.

8. J. F. Moran, "Aggression in the Health Care Environment: Part II, Theories of Aggression," *Healthcare Protection Management* 2 (1981): 8-15.

9. J. F. Moran, "The Officer and Aggression: Part III, Response and Responsibility," *Healthcare Protection Management* 2 (1982): 10-20.

10. K. Lorenz, *On Aggression* (New York: Harcourt, Brace and World, 1966).

11. S. Freud, *A General Introduction to Psychoanalysis* (New York: Boni and Liveright, 1920).

12. A. Bandura, *Aggression: A Social Learning Analysis* (Englewood Cliffs, New Jersey: Prentice-Hall, 1973).

13. P. H. Tannenbaum and D Zillman, "Emotional Arousal in the Facilitation of Aggression Through Communication," in *Advances in Experimental Social Psychology*, vol. 8, ed. L. Berkowitz (New York: Academic Press, 1975).

14. J. Dollard et al, *Frustration and Aggression* (New Haven, Conn: Yale University Press, 1939).

15. J. Altman, *The Environment and Social Behavior* (Monterey, California: Brooks/Cole, 1975).

16. A. M. Maagdenberg, "The Violent Patient," *American Journal of Nursing*, March 1983, pp. 402-403.

17. J. Viner, "Toward More Skillful Handling of Acutely Psychotic Patients, Part I: Evaluation," *Emergency Room Report* 3 (1982): 125-130.

18. D. Jacobs, "Evaluation and Management of the Violent Patient in the Emergency Settings," *Psychiatric Clinics of North America* 6 (1983): 259-269.

19. W. H. Anderson, "Psychiatric Emergencies," in *Emergency Medicine*, ed. E. W. Wilkins et al. (Baltimore: Williams & Wilkins, 1983).

20. H. M. Van Pragg, "Psychotropic Drugs in the Aged," *Comprehensive Psychiatry*, 18 (1977): 429-441.

21. W. R. Dubin, "Evaluating and Managing the Violent Patient," *Annals of Emergency Medicine* 10 (1981): 481-484.

22. J. R. Lion, W. Snyder, and G. L. Merrill, "Underreporting of Assaults on Staff in a State Hospital," *Hospital and Community Psychiatry* 32 (1981): 497-498.

23. J. H. Atkinson, "Managing the Violent Patient in the General Hospital," *Postgraduate Medicine* 71 (1982): 193-201.

24. R. W. Menninger, and H. D. Modlin, "Individual Violence: Prevention in the Violence-threatening Patient," in *Dynamics of Violence*, ed. J. Fowcett (Chicago: American Medical Association, 1971).

25. L. S. Lehmann et al, "Training Personnel in the Prevention and Management of Violent Behavior," *Hospital and Community Psychiatry*, 34 (1983): 40-43.

26. H. Pardes, "An Overview of Violence," *Resident and Staff Physician*, November 1982, pp. 60-70.

27. F. R. J. Purdie, P. Rosen, and P. E. Scott, "Prudent Handling of Patients Signing Out Against Medical Advice," *Emergency Room Reports* 3 (1982): 73-78.

28. E. S. Rofman, C. Askinazi, and E. Fant, "The Prediction of Dangerous Behavior in Emergency Civil Commitment," *American Journal of Psychiatry* 37 (1980): 1061-1064.

29. J. Kroll, and T. B. Mackenzie, "When Psychiatrists Are Liable: Risk Management and Violent Patients," *Hospital and Community Psychiatry* 34 (1983): 29-37.

30. J. P. Tupin, "The Violent Patient: A Strategy for Management and Diagnosis," *Hospital and Community Psychiatry* 34 (1983): 37-40.

31. G. Pisarcik, "The Violent Patient," *Nursing*, September 1981, pp. 63-65.

32. P. S. Appelbaum, A. H. Jackson, and R. J. Shader, "Psychiatrists' Responses to Violence: Pharmacologic Management of Psychiatric Inpatients," *American Journal of Psychiatry* 140 (1983): 301-304.

33. J. R. Lion, "The Biological and Psychosocial Treatment of the Violent Patient," *Resident and Staff Physician*, December 1982, pp. 33-37.

34. J. Monahan, "The Prediction of Violent Behavior: Toward a Second Generation of Theory and Policy," *American Journal of Psychiatry* 141 (1984): 10-15.

35. P. M. Fahrney, "The Secure Emergency Department," *Emergency Medicine*, May 15, 1983, pp. 40-49.

36. J. T. Turner, "The Role of the E.D. Nurse in Health-care Based Hostage Incidents," *Journal of Emergency Nursing*, July-August 1984: 90-98.

Chapter 5

Violence: The Child and Adolescent Patient

Anthony C. Zold, Ph.D., and Stephen C. Schilt, M.D.

JOEY AND "KERMIT": A PROBLEM

By 2:30, the ward secretary, two physicians, and two nurses from the Pediatric Ward all had called asking when I would show up to see Joey. I had received the original consultation request at 1:15. Joey was in a private room, and, curled in one corner of the bed, he looked younger than his six and one-half years. All I could see was a shock of unruly white-blond hair, two saucer-like, scared, blue eyes, and a huge, green Kermit the Frog clutched close to the little lump under the blanket. Joey's parents had divorced when he was one year old. His mother had severely abused him until he was five, when he was removed from her home and sent to live with his father. After a rough adjustment period, during which he seemed to fight constantly, Joey and his Dad were getting along beautifully. Joey was making friends and doing well in school. Then, Joey was diagnosed with cancer—Hodgkin's disease. The malignancy was rather advanced, but with extensive radiation and chemotherapy, he had better than a 50 percent chance of recovery. Talking as Kermit (Joey wouldn't talk to me, but Kermit was a great conversationalist), Joey was friendly, charming, and very lovable. But there was another side to Joey. He had injured three staff members on the ward. He bit one aide who was drawing blood, kicked a nurse in the breast, and broke another's glasses, causing only superficial scratches.

The staff was divided on how to handle Joey, and the disagreement had begun to degenerate into open conflict. During the previous week, the ward had lost three very young long-term patients; although two of the deaths were somewhat anticipated, the staff was deeply shaken. One faction wanted to, and actually did, provide more love, cuddling, comfort, and mothering to

Joey; the other wanted to, and to some extent did, establish more clear-cut structure, limits, rules, and punishments. Nothing seemed to work.

Meanwhile, Joey's father was confused and scared. At times, some staff members felt that he hampered ward efforts to manage Joey's behavior. He spent a great deal of time with Joey, consoling and playing with him, and he often offered to help ward personnel. When Joey refused to be taken to radiology, his father picked him up and carried him all the way. Talking to Dad alone, he could easily admit bewilderment, grief, anger, and an overriding sense of unreality.

OVERVIEW OF CHILD AND ADOLESCENT VIOLENCE

The management of Joey's violence was paramount to the staff, to Joey, and to his father. The issue, however, has far greater implications for the medical care setting. Although instances of violence by adult patients receive widespread publicity, violence is *most* prevalent among children and adolescents. Although five to twenty-year-olds made up only 8.5 percent of the population in 1975, of those arrested for violent crimes, 35 percent were under twenty.[1] Twenty-seven percent of serious crimes were committed by individuals under eighteen in 1974.[2] Since many instances of violence by children go unreported, these figures are an underestimation of the true incidence of childhood violence. For example, 34 percent of high school students in one study[3] admitted carrying weapons to school, and 25 percent of a middle-class, model student sample admitted committing acts of violence.[4]

Not only is violence more frequent in childhood, but in some ways, childhood violence is more difficult to handle in the health care setting. While caretakers would have little hesitation in calling for several security personnel to help subdue an out-of-control adult, they may feel more ambivalence toward someone like Joey. We would like to help, if we only knew how. We fall back on our preconceived attitudes, based on personal background and experience. Most of us believe we know how to handle children better than the average person (a statistical impossibility), and in the face of somewhat confusing scientific literature, we become instant experts. A random sampling of the recent literature on aggression and violence in childhood and adolescence stresses depression as the underlying cause and the direction toward which intervention efforts must be aimed; one study of aggression emphasized cultural and environmental determinants. One study stressed giving love and understanding, while another called for toughness and limits. Yet another talked in general terms of aggression being a symptom of something else.

One difficulty with studies of aggression is the lack of a clear definition of terms. Various authors consider somatic complaints, manipulation, causing accidental injury, violence for profit, anger fantasies, generalized rage, assertiveness, etc., as aggressive behaviors. This chapter does not make a distinction between accidental and instrumental (for gain) aggression, but focuses on behaviors which can cause pain or injury.

An imperfect, but helpful analogy to aggression in a medical setting may be high fever. Fever is a routine occurrence. It has different causes and various meanings. We need to understand its various causes, and we need to know how to diagnose and treat them; but we also need to be able to treat the fever itself until we identify the underlying causes.

This chapter reviews the relevant literature on the etiology of aggression in children; touches briefly on findings of programs designed to work primarily with the aggressive child or adolescent; and discusses the implications of childhood and adolescent aggression for the general medical setting.

ETIOLOGY OF CHILDHOOD AGGRESSION

Background

Attempts to explain the psychological development of aggression date back to the beginnings of psychology in this century. Freud at first theorized that the blocking of the libido caused aggression,[5] but quickly posited the existence of an aggressive drive.[6] Watson,[7] in his behavioral approach, challenged the drive theory and involved learning as the sole explanation of aggressive behaviors. Dollard's[8] theory dealt with aggression as a response to frustration. Bandura[9,10] introduced social learning concepts in stressing the imitation or modeling of aggression. Sears and his contemporaries[11] began careful studies focusing on the home environment of the child, including permissiveness and a high level of parental punitiveness contributing to childhood aggression.

Other early studies, Goodenough,[12] for example, focused on age and sex differences in determining stimuli eliciting aggression and the type of aggressive response elicited. Medical studies also have added to the list of potential etiologies of aggression. Common sense observations readily illustrate many of the theoretical positions. The enraged screaming of an infant, the temper tantrum of a spoiled child denied a request, the tough delinquent gang member, the abused child striking at others, the psychotic or intoxicated combative patient—all can be categorized into one or another theoretical framework. Treating aggression as a single, unitary concept, however, is an oversimplification. Studies that modify and specify earlier global findings that deal with sophisticated aspects of the area are generally more helpful to the hands-on health care provider. Ideally, one wants not just to know about "aggressive children," but to understand what types of aggression are manifested under what clearly defined and differing circumstances by which different types of children and what to do to prevent or reduce the aggression.

Psychodynamic Formulations

A number of psychodynamic theorists have modified Freud's original theory of the aggressive drive. For example, Waelder[13] theorized that a specific need for self-mastery and control is the crucial variable in the expression of aggression. This formulation is of interest because authors from different theoretical belief systems have also posited similar concepts as being primary in aggression. Maslow, among others,[14] stressed frustrations threatening specific ego functions, and Feshback[15] and White and Lippit[16] described aggression as an attempt to restore self-esteem.

Frustration and Aggression

There have been many studies indicating that increased aggression follows frustration, and that greater frequency or intensity of frustration may result in increased aggression. Other studies have modified or questioned this theory. Different types of frustrations may be more or less activating,[15,16] such as those relating to self-esteem. Other affective responses also may result from frustration, such as increased efforts at constructive play.[17] Also, stimuli other than frustration of an ongoing activity can lead to aggression; for example, pain,[18] anxiety,[19] dependency,[20] attention seeking,[21] and violation of expectancy and fairness[22] (such as not receiving an expected reward[23]) have all been associated with increased aggression. Studies demonstrate that certain children will respond aggressively to frustration, while others will not. For example, a study[17] showing that individuals with low ego strength respond aggressively found that those labeled over-controlled respond with increased constructive play when frustrated. Those high or low (but not in between) in persuasibility also showed increased aggression.[24] Two of the better studies in this area explored the interaction between the type of child and the type of stimulus that elicits aggression.[25,26] First, they address the question of whether aggressive children misperceive stimuli as threatening. Aggressive children were as accurate as nonaggressive children in identifying hostile and benign cues. Aggressive children actually gave more helping responses than nonaggressive children to the benign cues. The aggressive children, however, routinely misinterpreted ambiguous cues as hostile. The hostile, ambiguous, and benign cues were further subdivided based on whether they came from an aggressive or nonaggressive source. Both the aggressive and the nonaggressive children tended to ascribe hostility to ambiguous cues if the source of the cue was perceived as aggressive.

Imitation of Aggression

The imitation or modeling theory of aggression has received relatively consistent support.[27,28] Imitation of peers[29] and parents[9] has been demonstrated. There is more modeling of aggression if the model is reinforced for aggression, despite negative verbal labeling and description of the model.[30] Additionally, the increased aggression that followed a brief modeling experiment was evident on follow-up six months later.[29] Home environment, to be discussed further later, contributes to modeling. Decreased use of reasoning to manage behavior and decreased use of withdrawal-of-love techniques as punishment, especially with a hostile father or a rejecting mother,[31] increases the modeling of aggression. Reinforcement, to be discussed later, and personality factors also interact with modeling of aggression.

Reinforcement of Aggression

Direct reinforcement of aggression increases the likelihood of recurrence.[32,33] Intermittent reinforcement of aggression increases aggression more.[33] Patterson[34,35] showed the strength of peer group reinforcement of aggression. He also showed, however, that reinforcement increases aggression primarily for socially active, rather than noninteractive, children. Adult nonresponse to aggression may be a special reinforcer or disinhibitor for aggression.[36] It is known that a neutral response is seen as a negative reinforcer for children who are consistently positively reinforced and as a positive reinforcer for children who are consistently negatively reinforced. That is, children routinely rewarded for good behavior interpret silence as disapproval, while children routinely scolded for misbehavior will see silence as a sign of approval. Since aggression in children is usually negatively reinforced, it is likely that silence or no response from an observing adult serves to disinhibit or positively reinforce aggression. A breakdown or weakening of violence inhibition in some children has been attributed to the watching of violent television shows.[37,38]

Prosocial Behavior

A crucial area in the discussion of aggression that has been ignored by many authors is the development of moral judgment and the learning of such constructive prosocial behaviors as cooperation. This chapter will not detail the considerable literature on moral development, but briefly will stress findings on prosocial responses relating to aggression. Children who are neither reinforced nor have models for socially appropriate behaviors at home show higher levels of aggression.[39] Prosocial responses can be taught to children[40,41] through reinforcement[42,43,44] or through modeling.[45,46] The training of constructive behaviors reduces the incidence of aggression in experiments[34] and in real life.[42,43,44,45,46] In addition, when given a choice, children generally choose cooperative, task-oriented, positive responses over aggressive responses to solve problems.[47,22]

Home Background

Some of the previously cited studies referred to the background or home environment of the child. Low socioeconomic status (SES) of the family has been posited as an etiological factor for aggression in children in many studies. Yet there are some conflicting findings,[11] and social class categorizations do not represent homogeneous groupings. For example, there are demonstrated differences between urban and rural low SES children.[48] The biggest difficulty for the health care provider, however, is that SES differences do not adequately predict the potential for violence in a specific child or adolescent patient. Many children from low SES backgrounds are not violent, and many model children from middle class families do admit acts of aggression and violence.[4] More useful are studies exploring aggression in relationship to various home and parenting practices.

The three major dimensions of parenting that follow have been identified as relating to aggression in children: (1) permissive-restrictive; (2) consistent-inconsistent; and (3) affectionate-rejecting. Affectionate-rejecting is divided into two subtypes: cold and indifferent or punitive, with overuse of physical punishment. Studies that measure only one or the other of these dimensions have, to a large extent, found more aggression in children from permissive homes,[11] in children from homes with inconsistent discipline,[49] and in children from rejecting, punitive homes,[50,39] especially where high levels of physical punishment were administered.[51,52,53]

A number of contradictory findings to these results are a result of interaction effects among the dimensions. Some studies finding increased aggression with parental restrictiveness[54] did not factor out the effects of punitiveness, while lowered aggression with permissive parenting was only demonstrated in loving homes.[55] Generally, the least aggression occurs in children from warm, loving, affectionate homes in which the parents use firm, consistent controls directed toward the development of prosocial, more mature behaviors through the use of reasoning.[56]

Medical Factors

Studies on the environmental backgrounds of aggressive children provide general guidelines for health care providers. Medical literature furnishes additional clues about individual differences in violent behaviors. There are extensive reports on various neurologic etiologies of violent behavior, including anatomic, biochemical, physiologic, drug-induced, and electroencephalographic determinants. A neuroanatomic basis for violence has been well documented. The limbic system (specifically the amygdala and septal nuclei) plays a major role in aggressive behavior.[57] Interconnections between the hypothalamus and higher cortical structures also modulate responses. Biochemicals, including monamines, cholinergic agents, and serotonin are involved in mediating violent behavior, with norepinephrine playing a dominant role.[58] It has been suggested that testosterone may produce aggressive responses, and the marked increase of this hormone during adolescence correlates with an increase in violent crimes in this period. However, studies attempting to correlate testosterone levels with violent behavior produce conflicting results, and the etiologic significance is yet to be determined.[59]

Drug abuse is often the dominant factor in violence. The most common offenders are alcohol, amphetamines, hallucinogens (especially phencyclidine), diazepam, and cocaine. Withdrawal from narcotics, alcohol, and other central nervous system depressants can produce agitation and paranoia leading to violence. Drug toxicity can produce confusion and agitation leading occasionally to violent behavior. Narcotic analgesics, digitalis, phenytoin, and steroids are commonly prescribed agents with this potential. However, any centrally acting drug, including over-the-counter drugs with anticholinergic properties, may be involved.[60]

There has been much debate about the association of psychomotor epilepsy and violence. The evidence indicates that violence is generally not a manifestation of an ictal state,[61] but children with temporal lobe epilepsy have a very high incidence of interictal rage episodes.[62] The high incidence of electroencephalogram abnormalities among violent criminals is often cited, although such abnormalities at times may be the result, rather than the cause, of violent behavior.[63] A study of violent incarcerated adolescent males found 18 percent to have psychomotor seizures.[64]

Also described is the dyscontrol syndrome, which is characterized by "pathologic intoxication" resulting in violent acts and is often associated with EEG abnormalities.[65] This syndrome also is used to simply describe unprovoked, explosive episodes and is equivalent to what others have termed "explosive personality disorder."[63] There is evidence of the rare occurrence of limbic seizures resulting in violence, with neurosurgery alleviating the condition.[57] The evidence suggests that although neurologic factors play a role in violent behavior, they are only part of an interplay between psychological and environmental factors.

Other biological factors also may contribute. Various systemic illnesses and endocrine abnormalities can result in marked irritability and mood changes that may predispose individuals toward violent behavior.

Summary

This brief review of the literature confirms that complex and interactive factors are involved in the development and manifestation of aggressive behaviors. The capacity for aggression is inherent in the human organism. Physiological and biological factors, such as high arousal level, certain neurological and endocrine conditions, and some drugs, do increase the likelihood of aggressive responses. Environmental conditions and learning, however, interact with biology and play a crucial role in the development of aggressive behaviors. Children growing up in homes full of strife and rejection, who are randomly and inconsistently overcontrolled in a very punitive manner at times, and allowed inappropriate freedom in a cold, permissive manner at other times, are most likely to manifest numerous aggressive behaviors. When children are provided potent aggressive models, are reinforced for their aggressive acts and are not reinforced for prosocial behaviors, their aggressive responses are even more frequent and firmly established. Specific classes of situational triggers for aggressive responses that have been identified are frustration of an activity or goal; perceptions of being threatened, especially concerning ego functions such as self-esteem and self-control; perceived violations of expectations and fairness; feelings of anxiety, depression, or pain; vague and confusing situations; and the perceived lack of possible positive, prosocial response alternatives to a specific stimulus. The nature and intensity of an elicited aggressive response also depends on various interactive factors, such as past learning, the specific situation, and the age, sex, and emotional status of the child.

TREATMENT AND PREVENTION OF VIOLENCE

Introduction

During the childhood and adolescent years, most young people will have exhibited some type of aggressive behavior[4] under some conditions or situations. There are some children, however, who come to the attention of authorities for frequent and very violent behaviors. It is not the purpose of this chapter to review the extensive literature on juvenile delinquency, child abuse, or institutionalization issues such as the factors leading to violent riots. A brief look, however, at prevention and treatment measures aimed at this significantly violent population may offer clues for medical personnel on how to handle the occasionally violent child in the hospital setting.

Global Prevention and Treatment

Large-scale, general programs to prevent delinquency have not proven successful. The most ambitious of these, the Cambridge-Sommerville Youth Study, began in 1935.[66] Boys, aged five through eleven, were assigned counselors who met with the boys and the families and helped coordinate needed community resources. There were no differences in delinquency rates between boys in this intervention group and boys not assigned counselors, measured at the termination of the project in 1945[67] and at the 1955 follow-up.[68] Slightly encouraging was the finding that fewer of the boys with the most intense and longest interaction with their counselors became delinquents. Of concern is that more of the boys in the treated group had criminal convictions (and major mental illnesses) at the 30-year follow-up.[66] A replication of possible harm from an intervention effort was obtained in Hawaii.[69] Adult "buddies" were assigned to ten to seventeen-year-olds. Those with buddies who had not been arrested previously were subsequently arrested more often than those who were not assigned buddies.

The treatment of delinquents has generally been incarceration in a custodial institution. Recidivism, or treatment failure, traditionally has been extremely high—50 to 80 percent.[70,71,44] Establishment of a self-governing therapeutic milieu,[72] as opposed to a traditional, authoritarian approach, seemed to increase recidivism. Other therapeutic group home approaches[70] also showed little positive effect.

The disheartening results of the global prevention and treatment efforts are partially due to lack of specificity in the type of youngster treated and the approach used. There is strong evidence that there are various subtypes of aggressive children, that different therapeutic approaches have differing rates of success, and that different subgroups of children may respond differently to various intervention techniques.

Subtypes of Violent Children

A number of researchers[73,74,75,76,77,78] have identified major subgroups among delinquents. The three most consistent are the socialized-subcultural, the unsocialized-psychopathic, and the disturbed delinquent.

Socialized-subcultural delinquents (socialized aggressive) are likely to be accepted by their subgroups and generally involved in gang activities.

Studies[79] indicate that the socioeconomic status (SES) of the child's family is more a predictor for this group than for the other two. This group is also the least deviant in personality testing, although it has a somewhat lower IQ (especially verbal), and experiences less rejection from parents.[80,81] A comparison between delinquent and nondelinquent boys from the same high-delinquency area by the Gluecks[82] in one study and McCord[66] in another, however, did reveal family patterns contributing to increases in the 20 to 30 percent base rate for delinquency in the area. Overt deviancy of one or both parents, cold or rejecting attitudes toward the children, drastic family and financial situations, and lax or erratic discipline significantly increased the risk for delinquency. Mothers' love, however, was an important deterrent of delinquency in the socialized-subcultural group. Interestingly, in the McCord study,[66] delinquency was low with either the consistently punitive or consistently love-oriented discipline, and highest with the lax or erratic discipline.

Unsocialized-psychopathic delinquents (unsocialized aggressive) generally do not maintain close personal ties with others, seem not to profit from experience, routinely challenge authority, and feel that others are always unfair to them. Robins[83] has demonstrated that social class was less related to later delinquency in this group than in the socialized-subcultural delinquent group. Family disruptions also played a smaller role. Fathers' sociopathy and the number of antisocial symptoms shown during childhood were much better predictors of later problems in this group. Consistent, good discipline, however, was a positive mediating factor.

The disturbed delinquent belongs to a hodgepodge, heterogeneous group. Aggression in this group is almost incidental to other medical or psychological diseases or dysfunctions. This is the group in which aggression may truly be a symptom of something else.

Depression (masked depression) in children and adolescents is often manifested by aggression.[84,85] The presence of anxiety disorder (panic) or mood disorder (especially mania) increases the likelihood of violence.[60] Psychotic adolescents may show a high occurrence of violent behavior,[86] and paranoid ideation is frequently seen among violent offenders.[87] Attention deficit disorder with the usual marked impulsivity may be manifested by violent episodes.[85] Various personality disorders may cause an inability to cope with a change in environmental circumstances (such as hospitalization), and a violent response may be the result. Previously cited medical conditions also increase the risk of violence.

Success in treatment with this group is dependent on accurate diagnosis and appropriate intervention aimed at the underlying dysfunction.

Treatments

Immediate management of dangerous aggressive outbursts has been investigated in the medical literature, especially within this disturbed delinquent subgroup. Psychopharmacologic therapy is often useful in acutely controlling violent behavior. Whenever possible, drugs specific to the underlying disorder should be given. Benzodiazepines, such as Diazepam, are useful in alcohol withdrawal and may help reduce tension in the nonpsychotic, irritable, or impulsive adolescent. One must keep in mind side effects of respiratory depression and increased confusion with organic brain syndromes. Stimulants are effective in reducing aggressiveness among children with attention deficit disorder. Antipsychotics may also be useful in controlling violent behavior, especially if there is a thought disorder. Haloperidol is a good choice because it is less sedating. Lithium is also felt to have some antiaggressive properties; however, further studies must be done before its routine use for control of violence can be supported.[88] Propranolol has been found to control rage outbursts in children and adolescents with organic brain dysfunction.[89]

Different long-term treatment modalities also have been investigated and found to have differing rates of success with delinquents. As was seen, general approaches have been relatively unsuccessful. Additionally, client-centered and psychodynamic treatments also fared less well than behaviorally oriented approaches,[43] confirming previous findings that catharsis of anger, in and of itself, does not reduce aggression.[90] Marohn and his associates[91,92] use a theoretically psychodynamic approach in their work with violent adolescents, yet their success may be partially a result of their attention to behavioral detail. Marohn emphasizes immediate intervention to help the adolescent regain self-control and describes the routine progression from threats of violence to damage of property to physical assault if the signs of violent behavior are unheeded by the staff.

Generally, the more successful behavioral approaches focus on academic and social skills[44] and on family communications and contracting of responsibilities.[43] Studies[45,46] have also demonstrated that role playing and modeling of social skills not only increased skill levels, but also reduced recidivism in their samples. Additionally, Klein's[43] behaviorally oriented family intervention demonstrated that it may be successful in prevention if the target child is truly at high risk for delinquency. In that study, the siblings of the delinquents had a lower delinquency rate than that which was obtained in the control group.

Differential treatment programs for various subtypes of delinquents are rare. Sarason's[46] behavior modeling program, however, did produce better results with delinquents who were socially inadequate and immature. The

California Youth Authority classified delinquents according to Warren's[75,76] system and offered differential intervention based on the classification. Warren's system outlines concepts of interpersonal maturity and specific behavioral reactions. To some extent, behavior modification and transactional analysis succeeded differentially in some subgroups.[93] Most important, however, it was found that matching delinquent subtypes to staff members having coping skills appropriate to the subtype reduced recidivism.

Summary

The highlights of the literature on the frequently violent child indicate that generalized, supportive approaches neither prevent nor remedy delinquent acts. Ignoring, rejecting, or inconsistently dealing with inappropriate or aggressive behaviors tends to increase problems. Consistent discipline in a warm atmosphere and the training of appropriate skills such as communication and academics, through reinforcement and modeling, reduced later difficulties. Differential treatment of the different delinquent subtypes shows more promise than a general, across-the-board approach.

VIOLENCE IN THE PEDIATRIC SETTING

High Violence Potential

The previous sections highlighted the literature relating to the etiology and treatment of violence in children and adolescents. Given the findings, it is surprising that there is not more violence reported from the pediatric setting.

Violence-prone children are more likely to be injured and brought to a medical setting. Various medical conditions needing medical treatment have been associated with increased aggressiveness. Some medications themselves can increase violence potential.

The pediatric ward setting usually combines the vast majority of situational triggers for aggression that have been described in the literature. The child may feel depressed being away from home; anxious about what will happen; frustrated at restrictions on normal activity; upset over change; threatened in general, and especially threatened in terms of self-esteem relating to independence, self-control, and vulnerability; feel the unfairness of it all; be confused and bewildered from the ambiguity of not knowing what is going on and what will happen; experience pain, at times from caretakers who are supposed to make people feel better and who are models; perceive inconsistency from the caretakers as a result of shift changes and multiplicity of staff; and have almost no prosocial response behaviors available to solve problems. In situations of staff shortage or turmoil, feelings of rejection can occur from lack of attention or arousal from staff strife. If the staff's response to aggression is punitive or permissive, the likelihood of further violence is again increased.

Differential Diagnosis

As was seen in the previous section, the prevention or treatment of violence is most successful if it is applied differentially to different types of children and situations.

Differential diagnosis and differential description of the child's vulnerabilities, therefore, is crucial. Following the acute management of the violent patient, an appropriate evaluation must be done to determine the underlying cause. This should include a complete history, physical, and mental status examination considering a differential diagnosis based on the various organic, psychiatric, and psychosocial etiologies previously discussed. Depending on the findings, other investigations may be warranted. Blood and urine studies for metabolic and drug screening are often required. Neurologic studies such as electroencephalograms (EEGs) (awake and asleep, with occasional need for nasopharyngeal or sphenoidal recordings), skull x-rays, CT scans, CSF examinations, pneumoencephalograms, and brain scans may be required. Psychological testing may be needed to confirm a psychiatric disorder or clarify a subtle organic condition.

Multidimensional Intervention

In some settings, there are no provisions for in-depth diagnostic evaluations, and, even when there are, the evaluations can take a good deal of time. What is there to do until the differential work-up is complete? One successful approach is a combination of several interventions and may be best described as the shotgun approach. An analogy to this is found in James Michener's book *Hawaii*.[94] Michener cites an impending pineapple crop failure due to depletion of an unknown trace element in the soil. Extensive analysis had to be done to identify the missing trace elements, but to wait for the results would have been disastrous. In the interim, a fertilizer containing all known trace elements was applied to save the crop. In the pediatric setting one not only must provide a single intervention, such as warmth and caring, or structure and restriction, but all known preventive interventions in order to obtain healthy results. Multidimensional efforts are especially important with children, because their responses are usually not determined by a simple cause, but by multiple causes. Additionally, multifaceted approaches tend to unite pediatric staff members by eliminating disagreements over who is right or wrong, which can occur when deciding between alternative unidimensional interventions.

Intervention Guidelines

In establishing a multidimensional plan to prevent and treat violence in the pediatric setting, one must assume that all predisposing factors to violence are present and need to be addressed.

Assume a need for limits.

Provide a firm structure with routine and negative sanctions against violence; early intervention for behaviors that are precursors to violence, such as agitation, threats, and minor destruction, is crucial. Intervention must be calm and appropriate to stop behaviors. Ignoring the behavior will positively reinforce it.

Assume anxiety, depression, fear, and feelings of rejection.

Provide love, care, warmth, and attention in general, and specifically reinforce (and model) prosocial behaviors, such as appropriate communication of feelings, and mature, cooperative, and helpful actions. A transitional object, such as a teddy bear, is comforting at some ages and can be used for modeling appropriate responses.

Assume frustration of normal activity and boredom.

Provide activities, stories, and projects. The exclusive use of the "electronic babysitter" is risky.

Assume a threat to self-esteem, independence, and self-control.

Provide choices when possible, for example, the choice of drawing blood from the left or the right arm. Build in control, for example, by allowing the child to destroy the needle.

Assume tension and arousal.	*Provide* calm and relaxing atmosphere.
Assume confusion.	*Provide* clarity by explaining procedures, rehearsing what will happen, and showing the treatment room. Make sure the whole staff is operating from the same frame of reference. Take time to clearly inform parents how to reduce their confusion and anxiety. When possible, have one primary staff member be the caretaker for a given child on a shift.

The above list is somewhat general in nature. Each pediatric setting can specify additional concrete actions that suit its situation and patient population and make them available in written form. This list also needs to cover the eventuality that violence was not prevented. If violence occurs, the primary caretaker who has established a rapport with the child is the best person to try calm, but firm, talking in order to defuse the situation. Meanwhile, responsible authorities, including security staff personnel, must be notified in the case of adolescent violence. If restraints are needed, procedures for the use of physical restraints or medications (reviewed in the previous section) need to be delineated ahead of time to reduce confusion. Also, included on the list should be follow-up actions after violence. Not only must the violent patient be followed, but so must the other children who witnessed the occurrence and who are doubtless upset about what happened. Additionally, the written list must be reviewed periodically and after each occurrence of violence to see if certain preventible factors had been overlooked that could have helped calm the specific incident.

Developing and periodically updating the written plan for the prevention and treatment of violence is an important exercise in and of itself. The staff is brought together to work cooperatively, there is an increased sense of certainty about being able to prevent and handle violence, and many innovative approaches may surface that can be incorporated into a creative, growing plan of action.

Joey and "Kermit": Once Again

Joey is one example of multiple etiologies predictably leading to violence. He carried a number of predisposing factors, such as early abuse by his mother, which involved both rejection by a female and observing violence from a female; had lived in a neighborhood full of violence; and had a history of fighting. He was in pain at times, and had been given steroids, which, unknown to the nursing staff, can increase aggressiveness. Joey was scared, confused, and could sense his father's anxiety and confusion. His routine had been disrupted, he did not have enough to do, he had no choices about what happened to him, and he had no alternative behaviors appropriate to the situation. His emotional upset and his destruction of a coloring book had been ignored. The staff members did not communicate clearly among themselves, were upset over recent patient deaths, were pulling in different directions, and did not fully explain the procedures, plans, and prognosis to Joey or his father. His treatment was inconsistent—at times indulgent, at times overly restrictive. Kermit told me that one fight happened because somebody wanted to take him away from Joey to draw blood, another because Joey was going to be taken away somewhere "for good" (radiology) when his father was not there. His father would never be able to find him. The third incident of violence was an accident.

Consultation

The consultation request on Joey was handled primarily by a large, but brief staff meeting. All staff members, from aides to physicians, were included. They were told they did not need and would not receive guidance on how to handle Joey, since they already were aware of all the factors needed for a decision. The meeting's purpose was to express briefly the feelings experienced by the staff, to voice different goals in Joey's management, to advance plans and the reasons for them, and to consolidate different plans into a course of action. The feelings listed by the staff were anger, sorrow, frustration, and confusion. The goal in Joey's management was uniform. Everyone wanted the most effective care with the least upset possible. The plans for management were different, but the underlying premises very similar. The meeting quickly turned into a fun and exciting brainstorming session leading to consolidated courses of action. One goal of the plan was better communication among the staff members concerning treatment plans, side effects of medications, and other issues. One primary person was assigned to deal with Joey. Inappropriate behaviors would not be ignored, but dealt with immediately. Positive behaviors would be reinforced with extra attention and hugs. All procedures would be explained to Joey and his father. To make sure Joey understood procedures, staff members were to demonstrate on Kermit. When Joey had to be given shots or had to give blood, Kermit would say "Ouch, I don't like this. I am glad it's almost over," and, to Joey's great delight, would break the needle for disposal. Whenever possible, Joey (Kermit) would be given choices. Another goal of the plan was a written proposal based on these conclusions in order to prevent further problems and to avoid confusion should violence occur. An additional goal was to develop a written guide for patients and parents. In addition, before finalizing the course of action, the staff decided to elicit information from Joey and his father on aspects of care which troubled them.

Joey and Kermit: A Solution

Joey's father was delighted to be asked to assist. He had one suggestion that was incorporated into the plan. When Joey was to be taken to a new treatment area, such as radiology, it would help him to see the area prior to the procedure. Nursing staff did not have time to familiarize Joey with the area, but Joey's father did. Joey became more comfortable with the new surroundings and knew that his father would know where he was. His father could talk to him better about the procedures, having seen the treatment area himself.

Joey did not have any suggestions, but Kermit had two ideas that were accepted. First, Kermit was upset that his routine of having a snack of milk and crackers in the afternoon prior to his hospitalization was unavailable. Second, he never knew when staff members came into the room whether they were going to hurt Joey or be friendly and play and talk with him. Kermit received his snacks and was told that the staff members would wear a red baseball cap when they were coming to do a procedure.

EPILOGUE

In the six months since Joey and Kermit were in the hospital, the ward has experienced a significant reduction in the frequency of violent incidents. There have been no consultation requests about how to handle violent children or adolescents.

Joey's cancer is in remission. He and his father are doing well.

Thank you, Joey. Thank you, Kermit.

NOTES

1. F. Zimring, "Background Paper," in *Confronting Youth Crime: Report of the Twentieth Century Fund Task Force on Sentencing Policy Toward Young Offenders* (New York: Holmes & Meyer, 1978).

2. D. Mann, *Intervening with Convicted Serious Juvenile Offenders* (Santa Monica, Calif: The Rand Corp., 1976).

3. S. A. Cernkovich and P. C. Giordano, "A Comparative Analysis of Male and Female Delinquency," *Sociological Quarterly* 20 (1979): 131-145.

4. D. Offer, *Psychological World of the Teenager: A Study of Normal Adolescent Boys* (New York: Basic Books, 1969).

5. S. Freud, *Collected Papers* (London: Hogarth, 1925).

6. S. Freud, *Beyond the Pleasure Principle* (New York: Boni & Liveright, 1927).

7. J. B. Watson, *Behaviorism* (New York: People's Publishing Co., 1924).

8. J. Dollard et al, *Frustration and Aggression* (New Haven, Conn: Yale University Press, 1939).

9. A. Bandura and R. H. Walters, *Social Learning and Personality Development* (New York: Holt, Rinehart & Winston, 1963).

10. A. Bandura and R. H. Walters, "Aggression," in *Child Psychology*, ed. H. Stevenson (Chicago: University of Chicago Press, 1963).

11. R.R. Sears, E. E. Maccoby, and H. Levin, *Patterns of Child Rearing* (Stanford, Calif: Stanford University Press, 1957).

12. F. L. Goodenough, *Anger in Young Children* (Minneapolis: University of Minnesota Press, 1931).

13. R. Waelder, "Critical Discussion of the Concept of an Instinct of Destruction," *Bulletin of the Philadelphia Association of Psychoanalysis* 6 (1956): 97-109.

14. A. H. Maslow, "Deprivation, Threat and Frustration," *Psychological Review* 48 (1941): 364-366.

15. S. Feshbach, "The Function of Aggression and the Regulation of Aggressive Drive," *Psychological Review* 71 (1964): 257-272.

16. R. K. White and R. Lippitt, *Autocracy and Democracy: An Experimental Inquiry* (New York: Harper, 1960).

17. J. Block and B. Martin, "Predicting the Behavior of Children Under Frustration," *Journal of Abnormal and Social Psychology* 51 (1955): 281-285.

18. R. R. Hutchinson, R.E. Ulrich, and N. H. Azrin, "Effects of Age and Related Factors on the Pain-aggression Reaction," *Journal of Comparative and Physiological Psychology* 59 (1965): 365-369.

19. A. Ross, "On the Relationship Between Anxiety and Aggression in Nine-year-old Boys," *Dissertation Abstracts* 24 (1964): 5550-5551.

20. C. L. Winder and L. Rav, "Parental Attitudes Associated with Social Deviance in Preadolescent Boys," *Journal of Abnormal and Social Psychology* 64 (1962): 418-424.

21. E. K. Sanner, "Measurement of Aggression in Preadolescent Boys," *Dissertation Abstracts* 25 (1964): 4262.

22. L. Berkowitz, *Aggression: A Social Psychological Analysis* (New York: McGraw-Hill, 1962).

23. N. H. Azrin, R. R. Hutchinson, and D. F. Hake, "Extinction-induced Aggression," *Journal of Experimental Analysis of Behavior* 9 (1966): 191-204.

24. A. Roland, "Persuasibility in Young Children as a Function of Aggressive Motivation and Aggressive Conflict," *Journal of Abnormal and Social Psychology*, 66 (1963): 454-461.

25. K. A. Dodge, "Social Cognition and Children's Aggressive Behavior," *Child Development* 51 (1980): 162-170.

26. W. Nasby, B. Hayden, and B. M. DePaulo, "Attributional Bias Among Aggressive Boys to Interpret Unambiguous Social Stimuli as Displays of Hostility," *Journal of Abnormal Psychology* 89 (1980): 459-468.

27. A. Bandura, D. Ross, and S. Ross, "Transmission of Aggression Through Imitation of Aggressive Models," *Journal of Abnormal and Social Psychology* 63 (1961): 575-582.

28. A. Bandura, D. Ross, and S. Ross, "Imitation of Film-mediated Aggressive Models," *Journal of Abnormal and Social Psychology* 66 (1963): 3-11.

29. D. J. Hicks, "Imitation and Retention of Film-mediated Aggressive Peer and Adult Models," *Journal of Personality and Social Psychology* 2 (1965): 97-100.

30. A. Bandura, D. Ross, and S. Ross, "Vicarious Reinforcement and Imitative Learning," *Journal of Abnormal and Social Psychology* 67 (1963): 601-607.

31. A. Bandura, *Social Learning Theory* (Englewood Cliffs, N. J.: Prentice-Hall, 1977).

32. J. Davitz, "The Effects of Previous Training on Post-frustration Behavior," *Journal of Abnormal and Social Psychology* 47 (1952): 309-315.

33. R. H. Walters and M. Brown, "Studies of Reinforcement of Aggression: III. Transfer of Responses to an Interpersonal Situation," *Child Development* 34 (1963): 563-571.

34. G. R. Patterson, R. A. Littman, and W. Bricker, "Assertive Behavior in Children: A Step Toward a Theory of Aggression," *Monographs of the Society for Research in Child Development* 32 (1967): (Serial no. 113).

35. G. R. Patterson, "The Aggressive Child: Victim and Architect of a Coercive System," in *Behavior Modification And Families*, eds. L. A. Hamerlynck, E. J. Mash, and L. C. Handy (New York: Brunner/Mazel, 1976).

36. A. Siegel and L. Kohn, "Permissiveness, Permission and Aggression: The Effect of Adult Presence or Absence on Children's Play," *Child Development* 30 (1959): 131-141.

37. L. D. Eron, "Prescription for Reduction of Aggression," *American Psychologist* 35 (1980): 244-252.

38. W. A. Belson, *Television Violence and the Adolescent Boy* (Farnborough, England: Teakfield, 1978).

39. A. Bandura and R. H. Walters, *Adolescent Aggression* (New York: Ronald Press, 1959).

40. R. L. Updegraff and M. E. Keister, "A Study of Children's Reactions to Failure and an Experimental Attempt to Modify Them," *Child Development* 8 (1937): 241-248.

41. P. Brown and R. Elliot, "Control of Aggression in a Nursery School Class," *Journal of Experimental Child Psychology* 2 (1965): 103-107.

42. A. M. Horne, and G. R. Patterson, "Working with Parents of Aggressive Children," in *Parent Education And Intervention Handbook*, ed. R. R. Abidin (Springfield, Ill: Thomas, 1980).

43. N. E. Klein, J. F. Alexander, and B. V. Parsons, "Impact of Family Systems Intervention on Recidivism and Sibling Delinquency: A Model of Primary Prevention and Program Evaluation," *Journal of Consulting and Clinical Psychology* 45 (1977): 469-474.

44. H. L. Cohen and J. Filipczak, *A New Learning Environment* (San Francisco: Jossey-Bass, 1971).

45. M. J. Chandler, "Egocentrism and Antisocial Behavior: The Assessment and Training of Social Perspective-taking Skills," *Developmental Psychology* 9 (1973): 326-332.

46. I. G. Sarason, "A Cognative Social Learning Approach to Juvenile Delinquency," in *Psychopathic Behavior: Approaches To Research*, eds. R. D. Hare and D. Schalling (New York: Wiley, 1978).

47. M. Sherif et al., *Intergroup Conflict and Cooperation: The Robbers' Cave Experiment* (Norman: University of Oklahoma Book Exchange, 1961).

48. J. C. Madsen, "The Expression of Aggression in Two Cultures " (Ph.D. diss., University of Oregon, 1966).

49. J. Kagan and H. A. Moss, *Birth To Maturity* (New York: Wiley, 1962).

50. W. McCord, J. McCord, and A. Howard, "Familial Correlates of Aggression in Non-Delinquent Male Children," *Journal of Abnormal and Social Psychology* 62 (1961): 79-83.

51. L. D. Eron et al., "Social Class, Parental Punishment for Aggression and Child Aggression," *Child Development* 34 (1963): 849-867.

52. B. B. Allinsmith, "Parental Discipline and Children's Aggression in Two Social Classes," *Dissertation Abstracts* 14 (1954): 708.

53. A. H. Buss, *The Psychology of Aggression* (New York: Wiley, 1961).

54. E. J. Delaney, "Parental Antecedents of Social Aggression in Young Children," *Dissertation Abstracts* 26 (1965): 1963.

55. G. A. Watson, "Some Personality Differences in Children Related to Strict or Permissive Parental Discipline," *Journal of Psychology* 44 (1957): 227-249.

56. D. Baumrind, "Child Care Practices Anteceding Three Patterns of Preschool Behavior," *Genetic Psychological Monographs* 75 (1967): 43-88.

57. V. H. Mark and F. R. Ervin, *Violence and the Brain* (New York: Harper & Row, 1970).

58. M. Goldstein, "Brain Research and Violent Behavior: A Summary and Evaluation of the Status of Biomedical Research on Brain and Aggressive Violent Behavior," *Archives of Neurology* 30 (1974): 1-35.

59. B. Geller. and D. E. Greydanus, "Aggression in Adolescents: Aspects of Pathogenesis," *Journal of Adolescent Health Care* 1 (1981): 236-243.

60. J. H. Atkinson, Jr., "Managing the Violent Patient in the General Hospital," *Postgraduate Medicine* 71 (1982): 193-201.

61. A. V. Delgado-Escueta et al., "The Nature of Aggression During Epileptic Seizures," *New England Journal of Medicine* 305 (1981): 711-716.

62. C. Ounsted, J. Lindsay, and R. M. Norman, "Biological Factors in Temporal Lobe Epilepsy," *Clinics in Developmental Medicine* 22 (1966): whole issue.

63. J. H. Pincus and G. J. Tucker, "Violence in Children and Adults: A Neurological View," *Journal of the American Academy of Child Psychiatry* 17 (1978): 277-288.

64. D. O. Lewis et al., "Psychomotor Epilepsy and Violence in a Group of Incarcerated Adolescent Boys," *American Journal of Psychiatry* 139 (1982): 882-887.

65. J. Herskowitz and P. N. Rosman, *Pediatrics, Neurology and Psychiatry—Common Ground* (New York: McMillan, 1982).

66. J. McCord, "The Cambridge-Somerville Youth Study: A Sobering Lesson on Treatment, Prevention, and Evaluation," in *Practical Program Evaluation For Youth Treatment*, eds. A. J. McSweeny, W. J. Fremouw, and R. P. Hawkins (Springfield, Ill: Thomas, 1982).

67. E. Powers and H. Witmer, *An Experiment in the Prevention of Delinquency* (New York: Columbia University Press, 1951).

68. W. McCord, J. McCord, and I. K. Zola, *Origins of Crime* (New York: Columbia University Press, 1959).

69. C. R. O'Donnel, T. Lydgate, and W. S. O. Fo, "The Buddy System: Review and Follow-up," *Child Behavior Therapy* 1 (1979): 161-169.

70. R. Stephenson and F. Scarpitti, "Essexfields: A Nonresidential Experiment in Group-centered Rehabilitation of Delinquents," *American Journal of Corrections* 31 (1969): 12-18.

71. D. C. Gibbons, *Delinquent Behavior* (Englewood Cliffs, N. J.: Prentice-Hall, 1970).

72. M. Crafts, G. Stephenson, and C. Granger, "A Controlled Trial of Authoritarian and Self-governing Regimes with Adolescent Psychopaths," *American Journal of Orthopsychiatry* 34 (1964): 543-554.

73. H. C. Quay, "Personality Dimensions in Delinquent Males as Inferred from the Factor Analysis of Behavior Ratings," *Journal of Research in Crime and Delinquency* 1 (1964): 33-36.

74. D. R. Peterson, H. C. Quay, and T. L. Tiffany, "Personality Factors Related to Juvenile Delinquency," *Child Development* 32 (1961): 355-372.

75. M. Q. Warren, "The Case for Differential Treatment of Delinquents," *Annals of the American Academy of Political and Social Science* 381 (1969): 47-59.

76. M. Q. Warren, "*Classification for Treatment*," Presented at the National Institute of Law Enforcement and Criminal Justice Seminar on the Classification of Criminal Behavior: Uses and the State of Research, Washington, D. C., 1972.

77. C. S. Edelbrock and T. M. Achenbach, "A Typology of Child Behavior Profile Patterns: Distribution and Correlates in Disturbed Children Aged 6 to 16," *Journal of Abnormal Child Psychology* 8 (1980): 441-470.

78. T. M. Achenbach and C. S. Edelbrock, *Manual for the Child Behavior Checklist and Child Behavior Profile* (Burlington, Vt: University of Vermont, 1982).

79. L. McDonald, *Social Class and Delinquency* (London: Faber & Faber, 1969).

80. J. C. Brigham, J. L. Ricketts, and R. C. Johnson, "Reported Maternal and Paternal Behaviors of Solitary and Social Delinquents," *Journal of Consulting Psychology* 31 (1967): 420-422.

81. R. L. Jenkins, and A. Boyer, "Types of Delinquent Behavior and Background Factors," *International Journal of Social Psychiatry* 14 (1968): 65-76.

82. S. Glueck and E. Glueck, *Identification of Pre-Delinquents: Validation Studies and Some Suggested Uses of the Glueck Table* (New York: Intercontinental Medical Book Corp., 1972).

83. L. N. Robins, *Deviant Children Grown Up* (Huntington, NY: Krieger, 1974).

84. K. Glaser, "Masked Depression in Children and Adolescents," *American Journal of Psychotherapy* 21 (1967): 64-74.

85. R. Brumback and W. Weinberg, "Relationship of Hyperactivity and Depression in Children," *Perceptual and Motor Skills* 45 (1977): 247-251.

86. S. C. Inamdar et al., "Violent and Suicidal Behavior in Psychotic Adolescents," *American Journal of Psychiatry* 139 (1982): 932-935.

87. D. O. Lewis, "Delinquency, Psychomotor Epileptic Symptomatology, and Paranoid Ideation," *American Journal of Psychiatry* 133 (1976): 1395-1398.

88. M. Campbell, I. L. Cohen, and A. M. Small, "Drugs in Aggressive Behavior," *Journal of the American Academy of Child Psychiatry* 21 (1982): 107-117.

89. D. T. Williams et al., "The Effect of Propranolol on Uncontrolled Rage Outbursts in Children and Adolescents with Brain Dysfunction," *Journal of the American Academy of Child Psychiatry* 21 (1982): 129-135.

90. S. K. Mallick and B. R. McCandless, "A Study of Catharsis of Aggression," *Journal of Personality and Social Psychology* 4 (1966): 591-596.

91. R. C. Marohn, E. McCarter, and D. Linn, *Juvenile Delinquents: Psychodynamic Assessment and Hospital Treatment* (New York: Brunner/Mazel, 1980).

92. R. C. Marohn, "Adolescent Violence: Causes and Treatment," *Journal of the American Academy of Child Psychiatry* 21 (1982): 354-360.

93. C. Jesness, "Comparative Effectiveness of Behavior Modification and Transactional Analysis Programs for Delinquents," *Journal of Consulting and Clinical Psychology* 43 (1975): 758-779.

94. J. A. Michener, *Hawaii* (New York: Random House, 1959).

Chapter 6

Violence: The Geriatric Patient

William M. Petrie, M.D.

The elderly, especially in medical settings, are generally regarded as weak and helpless, not as individuals posing a risk of violent behavior toward others. Yet elderly patients are disproportionately represented in surveys of violent behavior. Medical illnesses are specifically responsible for reducing judgment and increasing impulsivity, and it is in medical settings that such individuals are encountered. It is also likely that, as the elderly comprise an increasing segment of the population in the next 50 years, larger numbers of violent elderly individuals will require attention.

Assaultive and violent behavior in the elderly is related to the underlying psychopathology of such patients; therefore, an understanding of the nature of medical problems that impair older persons' judgment and behavior will greatly assist in helping such patients and protecting those around them.

Much more attention appropriately has been directed to the elderly as victims, rather than as initiators, of violent acts. Particularly in domestic settings, the elderly have been frequent victims of abuse and violence. Medical practitioners have long been aware of the nature of this problem. In one survey, 60 percent of professionals reported weekly contact with abusive elderly individuals.[1] Abuse should be suspected in cases of unexplained trauma, neglected medical problems, malnutrition, and misuse of medication.[2] In many cases, little can be done by professionals, and the elderly victims themselves often reject help. It is possible, but unproven, that the elderly may ultimately respond to abusive and violent treatment with violence.

CRIME AND THE ELDERLY

Reports of violence by the elderly have been rare. The *National Law Journal* reports that not only is elderly crime increasing, but that it is taxing the criminal justice system.[3] FBI figures indicate that 400,000 felony arrests are made each year of people 55 or older, one-third of which are for violent crimes. Of those arrested, 25 percent are over sixty-five. The rate of crime among the elderly has increased dramatically during the last decade. A researcher for the Arizona State Corrections Department reports a 93 percent increase in inmates aged fifty-five or older in the years 1975 to 1980.[3]

It is unclear why there has been such a proliferation of crime in this age group, and it is more difficult to know how to deal with it. Many have suggested that the elderly are committing more thefts because of the difficulty in providing for necessities on their limited, fixed incomes. Others have pointed out that the elderly live outside of the mainstream of American life and feel alienated from the standards of the majority culture. Jails and prisons are not made for the elderly, with their special health needs, and the aged make extraordinary demands on staff time when they are incarcerated. For the aged inmate, jail may represent a life-threatening risk. The District of Columbia Correctional Facility was forced to establish separate dormitories and day rooms for older inmates. In general, older criminals are given lenient sentences, or no sentences at all.[3]

VIOLENCE IN MEDICAL SETTINGS

More than in other populations, the aged may more often present with violent behavior in medical settings, because of their frequent medical illnesses, which may increase their probability of becoming violent. The literature, which has been limited, indicates that violence is reported only in psychiatric patients. Tardiff and Sweillarn described assaultive behavior in 131 men and women over age sixty-five. Patients over sixty-five accounted for 14 percent of the total number of assaultive patients. These were generally first admissions to a psychiatric hospital, as opposed to repeated admissions.[4] In this sample, patients were referred to the psychiatric facility by medical practitioners or by nursing homes. Patients were overwhelmingly diagnosed as having organic brain syndromes. Men is this group were more frequently married and living with their spouses, while women were more likely to be widowed and living in group settings, mostly nursing homes.

In another report, those authors report violence being related to age, with assaultive and suicidal problems recorded in the youngest age groups as well as those over sixty-five.[5] Again, assaultive behavior in patients with organic brain syndromes was confirmed. The association of alcohol use with assaultive or suicidal behavior was not confirmed in this population, although prior studies have reported a strong association of alcohol abuse with violent behavior.[6,7]

Another recent report of violence in a hospital setting reviewed 29 incidents of verbal and physical aggressiveness at San Francisco General Hospital. Nearly all of the patients were mentally disordered, with impairment of impulse control and increasing tension. Of these, six had organic brain syndromes, nineteen were substance abusers, and three were delirious.[8] Because the elderly suffer from organic illnesses and delirium in disproportionate numbers, this study alerts professionals to the possibility of geriatric patients becoming violent in a general hospital setting.

One report[9] has been made specifically on violence in elderly patients hospitalized in a psychiatric unit. Two hundred and sixteen admissions to a geriatric psychiatry ward were surveyed for the commission of dangerous acts. This survey examined not just assaultiveness, but violent behavior of sufficient degree to represent a serious threat to the safety of others, most often to family and neighbors. Eighteen patients of 222 committed violent acts. The average age of these patients was 73.7. Most of these patients were males, and only a minority lived alone. Although this was a state psychiatric facility, usually associated with patients without financial means, more than 80 percent owned their own homes. Of these most dangerous patients, organic brain disease was diagnosed in 38 percent of cases; thus most patients (62 percent) were not cognitively impaired. These cognitively unimpaired patients were able to obtain guns, knives, and other weapons and to proceed with relatively premeditated acts. This majority did suffer from paranoid illnesses, but without clouding or impairment of consciousness. Hallucinations and delusions were common. Patients with a diagnosis of late paraphrenia[10] were the most violent. Their delusions were highly systematized, and their commitment to those delusional beliefs was high. In only one of 18 violent patients was there a documented history of violent behavior prior to age sixty.

Another group of patients in this study were aggressive, but not violent. Of these 222 referrals to the state hospitals, 121 had been aggressive. These patients were not nearly as dangerous as the violent group; threats, hurling objects, and striking staff or family members were their most common forms of aggression. Thirty-one percent of these patients were diagnosed as having senile dementia, while 23 percent had schizophrenia. Another 20 percent had either an atypical organic state or alcoholic dementia. Only 3 percent in this category had late paraphrenia. Of these aggressive patients, 34 percent were referred from nursing homes, 38 percent lived with families or spouses, and 28 percent lived alone. Disorientation significantly was associated with the aggressive group, rather than the violent group.

SUICIDE

Suicide is a form of violent behavior. Suicide rates increase with age, especially with male patients, rising from 22 per 100,000 in white males ages twenty to twenty-four to 52 per 100,000 in patients eighty and older.[11] Suicide is more common among lower class than middle or upper class males.[12,13] Suicide in the elderly has also been linked to social isolation, and marriage clearly provides a protective function for many. Most elderly suicides have no dependents and their contact with relatives is minimal.[12,14] Suicide is more common in urban than in rural settings.[14] Physical illness has been strongly associated with suicide in patients over age sixty.[14] Unlike younger suicide attempters, elderly patients seem more intent, using more lethal methods and succeeding more often.[15]

TYPES OF VIOLENT PATIENTS

Judging from the literature reviewed previously, knowledge of the diagnosis and etiology of violent behavior in the aged is a most valuable step in management and prevention. Of the psychiatric illnesses affecting the elderly, dementia, delirium, depression, alcohol and drug abuse, and paranoid disorders can all be accompanied by violence.

The Demented Patient

Dementia is a progressive, diffuse impairment of the cerebral hemispheres resulting in impairment of memory and cognition with accompanying personality changes. Slightly more than 50 percent of demented patients suffer from senile dementia of the Alzheimer type, an illness producing damage and atrophy to neurons in the brain. Violence by this group is produced by impairment of judgment, and is accompanied by confusion and loss of emotional control. Rather than planned, premeditated aggression, sudden impulsive acts emerge as usual social controls have been lost. Patients may strike at family or attendants if frustrated or confused. Memory impairment and disorientation are invariably present if the disease has progressed far enough. Families or staff members who have close contact with these patients can usually anticipate the frustrating or confusing situations likely to produce this behavior. Patients may be uncooperative and hostile when being bathed or escorted to unfamiliar locations. These patients almost always become worse when hospitalized because of the unfamiliar environment. Night is usually the time of maximal confusion, giving rise to the term "sundown syndrome." These patients follow an entirely new routine in the hospital, which includes trips to strange and frightening places (x-ray departments, operating rooms, treatment rooms), blood drawing, and constant intrusion by strangers (hospital staff). Consider the plight of the confused patient undergoing computerized tomography studies. The patients' heads or bodies will be thrust into massive modernistic machinery that they cannot understand. A response of fear and avoidance is normal.

Wandering is another problem with demented patients. In a confused or disoriented state, these patients may walk through rooms or corridors attempting to orient themselves. Rummaging through the rooms or belongings of others is not an act of theft or harassment, but may be viewed as such by their fellow patients, some of whom may be confused themselves. When demented patients do strike out, it will be with whatever is nearby, a cane, an ashtray, or a urinal.

Vascular or multi-infarct dementias more commonly result in confusion and a loss of emotional control, with deterioration at night.[16] This group of demented patients represents a potentially more explosive group than the patients with dementia of the Alzheimer type.

Occasionally, demented patients may verbalize, and even attempt to act on, suicidal impulses. Often, such patients experience catastrophic emotional reactions to their loss of awareness and control and feel they no longer want to live. These, like other aggressive acts, are sudden and impulsive. Unlike depressed patients, demented patients are rapidly changeable and may be in much better spirits soon after periods of depression and desperation.

The Depressed Patients

Depression is the most common emotional illness in the elderly, and its prevalence is greater in the presence of physical illness. Depression is common in patients referred to medical or surgical services in general hospitals and even more common in geriatric psychiatric units. In major depressive disorders, impaired sleep, loss of appetite, weight loss, hypochondriasis, and a lack of energy occur. In addition to these symptoms are feelings of guilt, boredom, and suicidal preoccupation. Paradoxically, the improving depressed patient may be even more likely to act on his suicidal feelings than those at the depths of depression. While younger depressed patients pose little risk to others, the older depressed patient, because memory loss and confusion are frequently associated with depression, may be more likely to show poor judgment and be aggressive and impulsive with others, most likely family or hospital staff members.

Alcohol Abuse

Alcohol and drug abuse in the elderly has long been ignored. Alcohol problems have been reported in up to 20 percent of some nursing home populations[17] and in 5 to 50 percent of outpatient populations.[18] In general medical wards, alcoholism can be found in the elderly at rates similar to those of younger patients. Surveys of Veterans Administration hospitals have noted alcoholism diagnosed in 20 percent of medical and surgical patients at one time in their lives.[18] Almost half of those patients were actively drinking at the time of admission.

Alcohol can produce violent behavior by three mechanisms: intoxication, withdrawal, and alcoholic dementia. Alcohol intoxication may produce impulsive feelings with accompanying reduced social judgment. As patients age, intoxication may more easily reduce judgment and precipitate angry or violent acts. Alcohol withdrawal consists of confusion, disorientation, and, at times, psychotic behavior from two to seven days following abrupt cessation of drinking. Patients in alcohol withdrawal are frequently disoriented and extremely confused. Paranoid feelings accompanied by violent behavior is common. Permanent cortical damage may result from years of alcoholism, producing a syndrome of dementia, memory disturbance, and agitation. We have found the patient with alcoholic dementia and a combination of impaired judgment, memory loss, and impulsiveness to be a potentially violent and aggressive individual, both in and out of a hospital setting.

Among hospital patients at a Veterans Administration medical center, alcoholics had a higher rate of attempted suicide, were more likely to live alone, and were more likely than non-alcoholic patients to be transient.[18] The so-called skid-row environment of some alcoholics carries an increased risk of violence and a particularly high suicide rate.[19]

The syndrome of alcohol withdrawal is likely to appear in general hospitals, while longer-term organic impairment that may lead to irrational, hostile actions is most frequently treated in a psychiatric unit or a nursing home.

Drug Abuse

Drug abuse by the aged is not widely recognized, and elderly drug abusers are frequently overlooked. Narcotic abuse by the elderly does occur, although quantities of drug consumed are reduced, and the elder users tend to shift away from heroin to morphine, codeine, and paregoric.[20] Abuse of prescription drugs occurs more commonly and surveys indicate that the chance of abusing prescription drugs increases with age for both men and women.[21,22] The chance for abuse is also increased by the number of drugs taken and the complexity of instructions; thus, hospitalized or ill patients will be at particular risk. Barbiturates and benzodiazepine tranquilizers are most commonly abused,[23] with Valium as the leading offender.[24]

While other over-the-counter drugs are also abused, it is the above-mentioned psychotropics that are most likely to cause confusional behavior, aggression, or violence. Withdrawal from both barbiturates and benzodiazepines results in anxiety and agitation, and disorientation and psychosis are possible in cases of barbiturate withdrawal. As patients become anxious, they may request drugs in the hospital; if refused, they may become fearful or angry.

The Paranoid Patient

Paranoid disorders have been associated with assault by adult patients, particularly by the elderly.[9] Although confused and disoriented patients may be transiently hostile or even paranoid, they are not true paranoids. This reaction is a result of their failure to remember or understand their current situations. There are two other groups of patients that present predominantly paranoid ideations, not accompanied by confusion or disorientation. One group is composed of schizophrenic patients who usually have been ill for many years and a second group of patients in whom the paranoid symptomatology begins in later life, for many after age sixty. It is also possible for some patients diagnosed as having manic-depressive illness to display paranoid symptoms.

The older schizophrenic patient is often housed in a psychiatric hospital. Some surveys indicate that more than one-third of long-term state hospital patients are diagnosed as schizophrenic.[25] In general or private hospitals, they are described far less frequently. These patients may harbor occasional aggressive or violent impulses, but the majority have predominant negative symptoms of loss of initiative, flat affect, decreased social skills, and withdrawal. For patients who have been on antipsychotic drugs for a long period, cessation of drug treatment may result in activation, increased psychosis, and an increased chance of violence.

For another group of paranoid patients, the onset of illness occurs late in life. Here a delusional state arises in a clear consciousness. Hallucinations and ideas of reference may also be present. This illness has been called late-onset schizophrenia or late paraphrenia.[10] Living in isolation may make these patients more paranoid. Their commitment to the delusional beliefs is strong, and they are more likely than younger schizophrenic patients to act on their beliefs.

Manic-depressive patients with manic psychosis are disruptive and present paranoid symptoms. Because of their expansive thinking, they will resist any attempt to restrain or hospitalize them. Even in a wheelchair, such patients may require several strong people to control them.

MANAGEMENT OF THE VIOLENT ELDERLY

An understanding of the psychopathology of the aged can reduce the risk of harm to the patient or others. As noted previously, the aggressive geriatric patient is likely to be quite different from other types of adult patients, and will require different management techniques.

The first principle of management is developing staff understanding of the origins of the patient's aggressiveness. This can be done through a series of in-service meetings with hospital, ward, or emergency room staffs. The goal of such meetings is to impart a general knowledge of the sources of aggressive behavior and review management techniques. The substantive knowledge in the area can be initially reduced to that which distinguishes the confused patient from the lucid patient. Staff can identify such patients by simple, initial questions, and once identified, it should be communicated from one staff member to others. Hospital staff should also have avenues to gain further information from physicians and nursing personnel.

The use of case-oriented discussions is particularly valuable. There should also be an opportunity for staff members to openly verbalize their feelings and responses to emergency situations or potential emergencies involving the violent elderly patient. Threats by older people may elicit much less decisive responses from staff members than a threat by an adult or younger patient. Feelings of fear are often unexpected responses in medical staff. In addition, once a patient has committed a violent act, the staff's anger with the offending patient must be recognized and accepted, rather than suppressed or expressed indirectly through neglect or avoidance.

> A seventy-nine-year-old patient had been hospitalized for nine years with a dementia associated with long-term alcoholism. He would forget where he was and assume he was home. Roommates and other patients were viewed as intruders and on occasion he would strike them suddenly. He never remembered his outbursts and at times was able to get along with others. Staff members reacted negatively to his outbursts and tended to view him as habitually aggressive and vicious, which eventually resulted in reduced staff contact and participation.

Staff members often minimize contacts with violent patients. Ironically, since the lack of current orientation is a primary factor in the aggressive behavior, reduced staff contact could easily result in increased disorientation, and in the case of this patient, an increased chance of future aggressive acts. If staff members had a better understanding of this patient's memory loss and impulsiveness as a result of a deterioration of his brain function, the patient could be handled with greater compassion and effectiveness.

Another problem occurring in long-term psychiatric hospitals is the placement of forensic patients, judged not guilty by virtue of insanity, back into geriatric units. This often occurs because the patients are judged not dangerous, but are unable to be released. Patients who have been tried for violent acts, including murder, stimulate fear and disgust in the staff even though the patient may have been hospitalized for 30 years or more. Staff members may require assistance in recognizing these feelings and coming to terms with such patients.

In more acute settings, staff awareness of alcohol and drug problems in the elderly may be helpful in recognizing withdrawal status and substance abuse confusional syndromes.

MANAGEMENT TECHNIQUES

The Confused, Assaultive Patient

This patient will come from a variety of diagnostic groups, including the dementias, delirious patients, and alcohol or sedative withdrawal states. Identification of the violent individual in this situation relies heavily on awareness of pertinent medical data. A physical examination, mental status evaluation, and neurological exam will identify various dementias and delirious states. Laboratory data will be able to confirm serious electrolyte abnormalities, renal failure, or hepatic disease which might produce an altered mental status. A social history will be indispensible in identifying patterns of alcohol or substance abuse, recent alteration in behavior, changes in social judgment, or behavior out of character to the patient. Even with this complete set of data, careful observation in the hospital by medical personnel will reveal emergent states such as drug withdrawal or increased confusion associated with adverse drug effects. Elderly patients who have had recent anesthesia or major surgery will predictably show periods of increased confusion and disorientation. Patients who have had cardiac surgery may also have periods of delirium and memory loss. The possibility of action toward others is reduced in these cases, however, because of the patients' bedfast or impaired physical capacities.

Correction of electrolyte abnormalities, treatment of drug or alcohol withdrawal, identification of drug toxicity, and diagnosis and treatment of the underlying medical problems will definitively solve most of these problems.

Management by other hospital staff will require some awareness of patients at risk for confusion and delirium and those with medical histories indicating a confused state. Identification of such patients by wrist tags or door signs, such as Complete Awareness of Patient Safety or C.A.P.S., will be of help.

Hospital staff will generally encounter these patients when their confused behavior is noticed by others. Reassurance and reorientation are the two most important principles in handling these patients. When dealing with such patients, staff should identify themselves and gently explain to them that they are patients in a hospital, that they are lost (if they appear so) and that the staff person is there to help them back. It is a mistake to assume such patients have awareness of their presence and actions until proven otherwise. Remember too, that many elderly may not hear well, particularly when in a frightening situation. It is not unusual for these patients to initially respond with hostility or demands to leave. Continued reassurance will therefore be necessary. A single staff person will usually be more effective than several, which may further frighten the patient.

Prevention of such assaultive behavior in the confused patient includes a program of reorientation, utilization of patients' existing faculties, and the creation of a familiar, comfortable environment. Patients should be reoriented and assisted before they become lost or confused. Families should be encouraged to bring pictures, familiar blankets, and articles from home to create a familiar bedside milieu. Calendars will assist failing memories, and large visible labels on the rooms of the patients will prevent embarrassing and disturbing cases of mistaken room identity.

Finally, such patients generally respond well to drug treatment. In one study of hostile patients with dementia, drug treatment was clearly superior to placebos in treatment of aggressive behavior.[26]

At 3:00 a.m., a ninety-year-old retired janitor awoke from his bed, and with an iron rod began striking objects in his house, destroying furniture and lights and threatening others. Police were called. They handcuffed him and put him in the back seat of a police car. He kicked the rear window out of the car and received an injection of an antipsychotic (thiothixene 10 mg) on admission to the hospital. On evaluation, he was totally confused and disoriented. He was fearful and imagined that he was in danger. In the hospital unit, he broke a door attempting to escape from the hospital ward, although he still was not aware of where he was. A neurological and psychiatric exam revealed a dementing illness with signs and symptoms typical of multi-infarct dementia. His behavior was controlled by reorientation, exercises, frequent reassurance, and contact and touching from hospital staff. Antipsychotic medication did not appear to be of significant value to him and was less helpful than personal interventions.

This patient's strength and fearfulness surprised police officers, physicians, and nurses alike. His fear and confusion were the driving forces behind his violence. When he was placed in a supportive environment, he became much more manageable.

The Paranoid Assaultive Patient

The paranoid assaultive patient differs from the confused assaultive patient by having a clear sensorium, the absence of confusion, and the ability to function in a more goal-directed manner. Diagnosis will be dependent on a careful psychiatric and social history. Patients may attempt to conceal the extent of their paranoia on direct questioning, and their psychotic symptoms may emerge in full only after hospitalization.

These patients, whether they are diagnosed as having schizophrenia, manic illness, late paraphrenia, or temporal lobe epilepsy, pose a more serious threat to others than than that posed by confused assaultive patients.

Awareness of patients' psychiatric status and history will be important for staff in addition to careful medical and psychiatric treatment, generally including antipsychotic drugs. Our experience with such patients led us to give them a "wide berth," avoiding confrontations or discussion of their problems in the acute phase. Delusions of this kind are not amenable to logic, and patients are extremely sensitive to imagined slights or even glances from others. In addition, it is difficult to predict when violence may erupt. Patients can be observed building tension, hostility, and defensiveness. When violent behavior does occur, it should be handled rapidly and with overwhelming numbers of staff members so that patients are not encouraged to resist. Nursing personnel and security staff will usually be needed to restrain such patients. The use of intramuscular antipsychotic medication is the most effective way to prevent harm to anyone involved. The use of three or fewer staff members to restrain patients may run a risk of agitating the patient even more. The more staff personnel used to restrain an actively violent patient, the less chance there is of harm occurring to anyone. We have observed that patients are actually relieved when, following a violent or aggressive outburst, firm external control is exercised over their behavior.

A seventy-eight-year-old retired businessman had been placed in a nursing facility because of a broken leg. At some point during his stay there, he became more garrulous and active and began preaching to other patients. He imagined that he was being abused by the staff at the nursing facility and that they were plotting against him to keep him from discovering a drug plot within the nursing home. Even though he was in a wheelchair, he struck one nurse with a cane and held several other patients hostage, not allowing them to leave his room. He asked family members to bring him a gun. They refused. Police were called, who transported him to a psychiatric facility. There, he was brought by police to the ward, but he threatened to hit or throw objects at anyone who came near. Although elderly and in a wheelchair, the patient was quite strong and fear-inspiring, screaming at the top of his lungs. Six nurses and security personnel were needed to subdue him for an intramuscular injection of 10 mg haloperidol. The patient ultimately recovered and was diagnosed as having manic psychosis. He was placed on low doses of lithium and ultimately was able to return to the nursing home.

This patient's activity illustrates the kind of violence likely to occur in an emergency room or psychiatric hospital. While the stereotypic view of a seventy-eight-year-old man with a broken leg would be of a harmless, frail man, this patient easily could have hurt an attendant or police officer. This case also points up the need to protect the patients themselves when violence erupts.

When guns or knives are involved, paranoid assaultive patients can be extremely dangerous as a result of a high degree of commitment to their delusional beliefs; that is, they wholeheartedly believe that their paranoid ideas are true and that they are in danger. They will often call the police or purchase firearms to protect themselves and they experience psychiatric hospitalization as a serious mistake, if not a further indication that they are being plotted against. They will resist hospitalization and may harbor paranoid thoughts weeks after treatment has been initiated. Their belongings should be searched thoroughly on admission (one patient brought a pistol to the hospital in his suitcase) and they should be isolated from dangerous objects in a hospital, such as silverware and sharp or heavy objects.

The Suicidal Patient

The elderly suicidal patient is usually depressed, but may be diagnosed as having schizophrenia, epilepsy, or no condition at all. Statistics indicate that the danger level of suicidal thoughts increases as age advances, particularly in white males. Alcohol and drug abuse may be accompanied by both depressive ideation and lowered impulse control, increasing the risk of suicide. Medical and nursing personnel should be aware of current suicidal thoughts as well as any past history of suicidal actions.

The major requirement in managing these patients is being aware of confusion or delirium and ensuring that confusion and demoralization from such a state does not contribute to suicide.

As with younger patients, it is also important to be aware of various degrees of suicidal tendencies in the aged, and dangerous objects should not be within reach of such patients. Antidepressant and antipsychotic drugs may both be of utility in medical management.

> A sixty-year-old, recently separated male had just recovered from a lengthy course of hepatitis. He developed secondary symptoms of depression and was hospitalized after initial attempts to return to his prior job had failed. He talked of his life as being meaningless and of having no purpose left for himself. He had a sleep disturbance and had lost 15 pounds. He complained of a memory disturbance and poor concentration. Security personnel noticed when he attempted to bring a knife back to his room from the hospital cafeteria.

Many of the positive risk factors for suicide found in the elderly are relevant to this patient's case, including recent medical illness, isolation, and the presence of a depressive syndrome. It is imperative that such patients be identified for all staff members and that cautions against suicide are made.

UNIT PLANNING

Unit planning should be able to accommodate all the situations described previously. In addition to in-service staff meetings, regular crisis drills may be useful depending on the profile of patients seen at that facility. A clear understanding of each staff person's role will greatly improve efficacy and safety, especially when subduing violent patients.

Newly admitted patients should be checked routinely for dangerous articles such as guns or medications, and should be prevented from gaining access to dangerous objects during their hospitalizations. A suicide awareness plan with varying degrees of surveillance should be available. For all elderly patients with neuropsychiatric problems, a brief mental status questionnaire should be given, the Kahn-Goldfarb Mental Status Questionnaire, for example. As in pediatrics, there are times when complete information must be gained from families. Where appropriate, a social worker or other professional should be available to take this information on admission.

In geriatric services, a ward milieu providing support for confused and disoriented patients should be available to prevent increased confusion. For brief periods of time, reorientation improves cognitive function; moreover, such an environment provides comfort and security for the patient. The orientation materials (calendars, newspapers, etc.) are inexpensive; staff time to spend with patients will be the most important expenditure.

SUMMARY

Elderly patients may be more violent than other adult patients because of their impaired judgment and tendency toward actions that occur as a part of many geriatric illnesses, particularly neuropsychiatric disorders. Patients with dementia, delirium, and degenerative central nervous system diseases may become violent or assaultive as a result of their confusion and memory loss. Such assaultiveness usually can be predicted and is much less dangerous because of the disorganization of the patients's thinking and activities. Prevention may be aimed at creating a more comforting, reassuring environment for these frightened, confused patients. Another group of patients are diagnosed as having schizophrenia, late paraphrenia, and manic illnesses. Their acts are more dangerous and less predictable than those of the former group, but these patients often respond well to antipsychotic drugs. Finally, suicide is an act of violence particularly common among elderly white males. Hospital staff should be able to assess suicidal potential and protect patients from themselves.

Medical settings must provide the ability to understand the sources of violent behavior in the elderly and to reduce the risks to the population at large while they serve the medical needs of the aged.

NOTES

1. T. Hickey & R. L. Douglass, "Mistreatment of the Elderly in the Domestic Setting: An Exploratory Study," *American Journal of Public Health* 71 (1981): 500-507.

2. T. A. O'Malley et al., "Identifying and Preventing Family-mediated Abuse and Neglect of Elderly Persons," *Annals of Internal Medicine* 98 (1983): 998-1005.

3. National Law Journal, An Elderly Crime Wave (Vol. 4, #39), 1982.

4. K. Tardiff & A. Sweillam, "The Occurrence of Assaultive Behavior Among Chronic Psychiatric Inpatients," *American Journal of Psychiatry* 139 (1982): 212-215.

5. K. Tardiff & A. Sweillam, "Assault, Suicide and Mental Illness," *Archives of General Psychiatry* 37 (1980): 164-169.

6. C. E. Climent & F. R. Ervin, "Historical Data in the Evaluation of Violent Subjects," *Archives of General Psychiatry* 27 (1972): 621-624.

7. F. G. Johnson, B. G. Frankel, and R. G. Ferrence, "Self-Injury in London, Canada: A Prospective Study," *Canadian Journal of Public Health* 66 (1975): 307-316.

8. H. N. Ochitill and M. Krieger, "Violent Behavior Among Hospitalized Medical and Surgical Patients," *Southern Medical Journal* 75 (1982): 151-155.

9. W. M. Petrie, E. C. Lawson, & M. H. Hollender, "Violence in Geriatric Patients," *Journal of the American Medical Association* 248 (1982): 443-444.

10. M. D. Hubert & S. Jacobson, "Late Paraphrenia," *British Journal of Psychiatry* 113 (1967): 461-469.

11. National Center for Health Statistics, *Vital Statistics of the United States, 1976, Mortality* (Washington, D.C.: U.S. Government Printing Office, 1979).

12. E. W. Bock & I. L. Webber, "Social Status and the Relational System of Elderly Suicides," *Life-threatening Behavior* 2 (1972): 145-159.

13. J. M. A. Weiss, "Suicide in the Aged," in *Suicidal Behaviors,* ed. H. L. P. Resnik (Boston: Little, Brown, 1968).

14. P. Sainsburg, "Social and Epidemiological Aspects of Suicide with Special Reference to the Aged," in *Processes of Aging: Social and Psychological Perspectives,* vol. 2, R. H. Williams, C. Tibitts, & E. Donahue eds. (New York: Atherton, 1963).

15. W. Breed & C. L. Huffine, "Sex Differences in Suicide Among Older White Americans: A Role and Developmental Approach," in, *Psychopathology of Aging,* O. J. Kaplan ed. (New York: Academic Press, 1979).

16. V. C. Hachinski et al., "Cerebral Blood Flow in Dementia," *Archives of Neurology* 32 (1975): 632-637.

17. P. Graux, "Alcoholism of the Elderly," *Review Alcoholism* 15 (1959): 46-48.

18. M. A. Shuckit & P. A. Pastor, "Alcohol-related Psychopathology in the Aged," in *Psychopathology of Aging,* ed. O. J. Kaplan (New York: Academic Press, 1979).

19. D. J. Bouge, *Skid Row in American Cities* (Chicago: Community and Family Study Center, University of Chicago, 1963).

20. W. C. Capel & G. T. Stewart, "The Management of Drug Abuse in Aging Populations: New Orleans Findings," *Journal of Drug Issues* 1 (1971): 114-120.

21. M. J. Abrahams, J. Armstrong, & F. A. Whitlock, "Drug Dependence in Brisbane," *Medical Journal of Australia* 2 (1970): 397-404.

22. A. George, "Survey of Drug Use in a Sydney Suburb," *Medical Journal of Australia,* 2 (1972): 233-237.

23. E. F. Pascarelli, "Drug Dependence: An Age-old Problem Compounded by Old Age," *Geriatrics* 29 (1974): 109-115.

24. D. M. Petersen & C. W. Thomas, "Acute Drug Reactions Among the Elderly," *Journal of Gerontology* 30 (1975): 552-556.

25. I. N. Mensk, "The Older Schizophrenic," in *Psychopathology of Aging,* ed. O. J. Kaplan (New York: Academic Press, 1979).

26. W. M. Petrie et al., "Loxapine in Psychogeriatrics: A Placebo and Standard Controlled Clinical Investigation," *Journal of Clinical Psychopharmacology* 2 (1982): 122-127.

Chapter 7

Violence: The Drug/ Alcohol Patient

Dwayne Piercy, Ph.D.

Violence is generally defined as a forceful act or threat, the intent of which is to injure, damage, maim, or destroy some person or object. Such an act may include murder, rape, assault, vandalism, or a variety of other actions defined by society as undesirable and unacceptable behavior. Even the mere existence of these acts is frightening to each of us as individuals and threatens us by raising the possibility that such actions may eventually affect us personally, rather than abstractly.

In recent years, the FBI's *Uniform Crime Reports* have aroused in many of us the fear that we are closer than ever to actually experiencing violence on a very personal level. Expanded police agencies with increasingly sophisticated methods of statistical data analysis receive widespread coverage by the media. This, along with reports of rising crime rates, has engendered a more focused awareness that violence is a growing part of our society.

Whether this increase in violence is a reflection of increased efficiency in data acquisition or a natural consequence of such factors as increased population and urbanization is not of any great concern to the average person. The concern of most individuals is much more visceral: "Why does violence happen? Can it happen to me? Can I prevent it?" For those employed in clinical settings, especially in settings that deal with emergent conditions, the concerns tend to be at least as visceral as those of the average citizen: "Why do the patients I encounter sometimes become violent? Will I be the object of this violence? How can I minimize my risk?"

In examining these very real concerns, it is, as usual, the "Why?" questions that elicit the most academic and involved answers. The search for an explanation of the violent aspects of human behavior is long and involved. Arguments for causation have been advanced to support theories that are phylogenetic, political, moral, racial, economic, morphological, sociological, environmental, familial, marital, biochemical, naturalistic, theological, ritualistic, and cultural. None of these theories fully can explain all behavior.

123

Almost certainly, no one theory adequately will explain causation in any one situation or incident. We are concerned with human behavior, and such behavior tends to have multiple, not single, causation.

Any extended examination of the violence in our society today will result in the finding that the use of alcohol or other chemical agents is an important component of many acts of violence and crime.[1,2,3] Nicol et al.[4] in Great Britain and Mayfield[5] in the United States found violent prisoners to be alcoholic in about one-third of the cases examined. Mayfield also noted that the majority of the prisoners in his study were intoxicated at the time of their violent acts. In an examination of the factors involved in family violence, Viken[6] noted that the literature supports the idea of a relationship between alcohol abuse by the husband and the battering of his wife, although this relationship shows a wide range of reported incidence. Byles[7] found that acts of physical violence are more than twice as likely to occur in families with alcohol problems as in families without such problems. The targets of the violence are usually the nonalcoholic spouse and children. The connection between death and injury in automobile accidents and alcohol intoxication is both well known and widely discussed.[8]

In a review of the literature concerning the influence of drug abuse and alcoholism on the incidence of child abuse, Sarles[9] found that opinions on the subject varied considerably. However, most workers in the field of substance abuse find it useful to inquire about child abuse because it is so frequently observed in their caseloads, whatever the statistics of a particular study may suggest. Perhaps one of the strongest opinions concerning the type of child abuse more specifically labeled as incest between an adult and a child is that of Meiselman,[10] who concludes that as many as 75 percent of adult incest perpetrators are alcoholic.

In a study dealing with an investigation of the utility of a situational approach to violence, Steadman[3] collected data on violence from 534 persons in Albany County, New York. He interviewed a sample of persons carefully chosen to be representative of the general population of the area, a sample of former mental patients who had lived in the community for one year or longer, and a sample of ex-offenders who had resided in the community at least six months.

One of the many interesting findings of this study was that, for all sample groups, as the severity of the dispute (and hence the degree of violence) increased, the likelihood that the violence occurred in bars and outdoor locations increased. Disputes involving weapons and hitting tended to occur between 9 p.m. and 6 a.m.—prime bar times. As might be expected, the data showed that the more severe disputes tended to involve alcohol and drug use. This finding was particularly true among the ex-offender group members and their antagonists.

An interesting confirmation of the relationship between violence and chemical abuse comes from a study in South Africa by Hemphill and Fisher.[11] Their subjects were 604 males who had been sent by the courts for psychiatric evaluation. The authors found that 52 percent of their patients were habitual users of drugs (including alcohol). They also discovered that alcohol, especially, was often associated with violent behaviors, while marijuana was not. Similar findings were reported in a series of studies by Tinklenberg.[12,13,14] Subjects in these studies were male juvenile offenders under the jurisdiction of the California Youth Authority. The results of these studies tended to confirm those just cited by Hemphill and Fisher,[11] that alcohol was the drug most often found associated with crimes involving either physical or sexual violence, while cannabis (marijuana) was found much less often, and, indeed, was noted by the subjects to have a calming effect upon them.

Further review of both popular and scientific literature leaves little doubt that ours is a society with a great deal of violence, and that acts of violence are often associated with the use of drugs, especially that most readily available and seriously abused of drugs: alcohol. This conclusion was underscored in an article in *Time* magazine by Anderson,[15] who took note of the prevalence of drug dependency among wife beaters, rapists, and child abusers. And it is probably no coincidence that in street riots, such as the racial riots of the 1960s, one of the most frequent targets of the rioters was the neighborhood liquor store.

DRUG USE AND VIOLENCE IN THE HEALTH CARE SETTING

Health care settings are actually small communities, whether they are emergency rooms, psychiatric wards, general hospitals, or free-standing clinics. They bring together small numbers of the general population on a more selective basis. However, they tend to be largely reflective of their referent society. If the environment about them is English-speaking, they tend to be English-speaking. If the society about them tends to be Judaeo-Christian, they tend to be Judaeo-Christian. Similarly, if the society they serve tends to have incidences of acts of violence, they also tend to experience such acts. Health care settings, therefore, might be expected to experience a number of violent acts for several reasons. The suicidal client is more often delivered to a hospital emergency room than to a jail. The number of states with uniform intoxication acts has mandated an increase in the number of chemical abusers who are delivered to emergency rooms or state or private hospitals, rather than to places of incarceration. Increasing emphasis on the rights of patients in health care settings has restricted the use of routine room searches in psychiatric hospitals. There has been a great shift to the evaluation of alcohol abuse in more disease-oriented terms than in past years, when the emphasis was on more moralistic explanations. The result of this shift in thinking is that alcohol and drug abusers are brought to the health care facility for treatment more frequently than ever before.

With these myriad societal changes, a greater incidence of violence associated with drug use may be expected in such facilities, either because violent drug abusers are brought in for treatment of the drug-violence connection, or because they abuse drugs while already in such settings. There is now considerable evidence that personnel in emergency rooms, hospitals, and other health care settings are frequent targets for assaults by patients.[16,17,18,19,20,21,22] Particularly alarming are the findings of Whitman et al.[23] that more than a third of the psychiatrists in their survey had been assaulted by a patient within a one-year period. Similarly, Madden et al.[24] discovered that nearly half of the respondents in their study had been assaulted by a patient at some point in their careers.

There is also evidence[25] that more than half of the patients reviewed in one study of violence in emergency rooms had consumed alcohol before their aggressive actions occurred. The same authors also concluded in a series of studies[25,26,27] that alcohol intoxication had been a factor in as many as one-fourth of cases of violence involving psychiatric patients.

Even if such evidence did not exist, health care professionals are well aware of the risks of encountering violent patients, and many practitioners seek to protect themselves from risk by avoiding such patients entirely. This is well illustrated by Tardiff,[28] who conducted a survey of psychiatrists in the Boston area on their work with violent patients. He found that less than half of those questioned evaluated or treated such patients, and that those who did tended to be less than forty years old and were often still receiving training. This suggests that more experienced psychiatrists prefer to pursue careers in which they avoid such patients.

Given the distinct possibility of violence in health care settings, it is certainly tempting to try to avoid psychiatry or emergency room duty and thus evade violent patients, particularly those who have been drinking or using drugs. There are, however, many reasons that this step is not practical. For both legal and practical reasons, it is frequently necessary for staff members to carry out their duties with potentially violent, drug-influenced persons. As already noted, many states have uniform intoxication acts requiring that intoxicated persons be transported to health care facilities for mandatory treatment in lieu of incarceration. Probably the majority of medical care staffs and their administrators prefer to offer such services, possibly for humanitarian reasons, but more likely to conform with laws and community expectations. Obviously, most reasonable citizens would prefer to have a relative with drug-induced problems hospitalized, and most reasonable health care managers would prefer to have a minimum of police officers on the wards and in the emergency rooms of their facilities if they oblige these community preferences.

Health care professionals who contemplate avoiding drug abusers and potentially violent patients should be aware that those patients already may be present on medical and surgical wards. This point is implied in a study by Ochitill and Krieger,[29] who investigated 29 incidents of violent behavior among the 350 medical and surgical patients of a general hospital. These incidents occurred within a two-year span of time. In this subgroup of 29 violent patients, 19 were diagnosed as substance abusers. The authors also noted that, during the time their study was conducted, approximately 15 percent of the patients in the medical and surgical units of their hospital were diagnosed on discharge as having some indication of drug-related problems.

Granted that health care workers in a variety of settings will come in contact with substance-abusing and potentially violent patients, it is to their advantage to develop the knowledge and skills necessary to distinguish between those situations in which they can reasonably intervene and those in which it is best for them to abandon a treatment stance for a more security-based approach. For their own safety and peace of mind, they should develop a substantial repertoire of preventive strategies for use with the potentially violent individual in order to supplement and supersede the sometimes excessively reactive behaviors that tend to be the primary preoccupation of some health care training and staff-development programs.

In 1974, the American Psychiatric Association reviewed the available information on the ability of the psychiatric profession to accurately predict whether or not a person would become violent or dangerous. It concluded that such predictions were unreliable and lacked true validity.[30] In the ten years since that report, extensive research into violence has yielded considerable statistical and empirical data about violence,[3] but that data seems to have resulted in only minor improvements in the ability of the clinician to anticipate violence in patients. Nevertheless, the clinician continues to be called on to make this prediction and to manage the violent individual in a just, humane, and legal manner.

Probably the best advice on dealing with the potentially or actually violent individual under the influence either of alcohol or other drugs is that of Marjot: "Unless there is an overriding duty either as a citizen or as a doctor it is best to avoid becoming involved with someone who is actually or potentially violent."[31] This author also points out that the police are or should be better prepared to handle such persons. Unfortunately, there are many situations in which health care staff members are required to deal with potentially violent, drug-influenced individuals. For both legal and administrative reasons, staff members must carry out their duties with such persons.

There are many important factors that influence the drug abuser to exhibit violence in the health care setting. Proper early identification of such factors is important in anticipating such violent behavior. For the health practitioner, the circumstances surrounding the arrival of the individual at the health care facility are a prime consideration and should be assessed immediately. Is the person there voluntarily? Is the person asking for help? Or has the individual been forced to come in by family, friends, or authorities? As a rule of thumb, the more willing the patient is to seek help, the less potential for violence. A major exception is when the abuser asks for a type of help with which the provider might not agree, for example, the dispensing of narcotics to an addict. This exception may occasion an immediate confrontational situation.

The type of health care setting itself is quite important. Is it equipped to deal adequately with the potentially violent drug abuser? Is it adequately staffed with additional personnel in easy reach of the violent situation? Is it a place where the potentially violent person can feel secure, or is it a place where the person may be led to feel even more threatened?

The health care settings in which violence occurs can be quite varied, and each has its potential problems. Such violence may occur in the general hospital setting,[32,33] in the therapeutic community,[34] in the physician's private office,[24] or in the emergency room.[27] All of these locations have characteristics that can either increase or decrease the probability for violence, and these should be considered in management of the violent patient. As well, each unique setting may have its own written guidelines related to preventing and dealing with the violent patient.

It is very important for the health care worker to know who is accompanying the individual. Is it a police officer, minister, angry wife, or supportive friend? All have different implications for the genesis of violence and for its prevention. It is the practitioner's task to assess these implications.

Of empirical importance is the nature of the violence itself. Is it a suicidal attempt? Does it involve assault on another person with or without weapons or provocation? Is the violent action specific and goal-directed, or is it generalized and random? Efforts to manage an attempt at suicide will be much different than efforts to manage generalized violence. The former may require an additional assessment for depression, while the latter may require an evaluation for a medical condition underlying the more apparent drug condition.

The final two factors are the most difficult to assess and take the most time and effort: the type of drugs involved and the type of person using the drugs.

Common Drugs of Abuse

Violence associated with chemical abuse tends to occur in a particular stage of that abuse: during intoxication, during withdrawal, or in what might be called the residual stage of abuse. Since different drugs have different implications for anticipating violence, it is most important to identify the drug involved immediately. It is important to know if it is a street drug, an over-the-counter preparation, or a prescribed drug, since this can give information about the purity of the drug. Once the drug is known, added potential for predicting violence exists.

The first stage in drug abuse is intoxication. This is the period in which the so-called toxicomanic symptoms may occur. Here, the person is most directly and strongly affected by the drug itself. This phase may last for varying lengths of time, but it endures as long as the drug is actively consumed and for a defined period afterward, depending on such factors as the type and quality of the drug consumed, its mechanisms of action in the body, and the health condition, age, degree of habitation, physical environment, and the social milieu of the user.

The second stage of drug abuse is the period of withdrawal, or discontinuation of the drug. Depending on the drug and other factors, symptoms may be mild or severe, and behavior may become quite dramatic with great potential for violence. Examples would include the behaviors associated with heroin withdrawal so well depicted in movies and on television, and the tremors, seizures, and delirum tremens (d.t.'s) of alcohol withdrawal. Less dramatic examples would include the irritability following withdrawal from tobacco or caffeine.

The final phase in drug abuse may be termed the residual stage. Here are grouped the long-term conditions sometimes found after extended periods of drug dependency and misuse. One example with potential for violence is the organic brain syndrome which follows years of drug use and may include physical, mental, and emotional debilitation. Another example would be dementia associated with alcoholism and diagnosed no sooner than three weeks after discontinuing alcohol use.[35]

Almost any drug can have negative properties if improperly administered or ingested. Even water consumed in large amounts can lead to increasingly psychotic symptomatology, especially in schizophrenic patients. Such conditions then have the potential for violence. However, mind-altering drugs are the most frequent sources of violence in most health care settings. Support for this conclusion is supplied by the National Commission on Marijuana and Drug Abuse.[36] In 1973, after reviewing and summarizing the research available on the relationship between violence and drug abuse, the commission found evidence of a relationship between violence and alcohol, barbiturates, and amphetamines. Simonds and Kashani[37] interviewed 112 delinquent males in a training school to investigate the relationship between specific drugs and violence. They found a positive relationship between crimes committed against persons and five drugs: amphetamines, phencyclidine (PCP), barbiturates, cocaine, and diazepam (Valium). They also found a connection between crimes committed against property and five drugs: cocaine, alcohol, heroin, marijuana, and LSD.

It is not possible here to review every drug of abuse associated with violence, but I will review those drugs most frequently cited in connection with violence in the literature and in my clinical experience. One additional drug, lithium carbonate, also will be cited because of its increasing use in health care settings, and some of the problems observed with it. Finally, the occurrence of violence in the presence of mixed drugs is also discussed. Considered in general terms, the drugs most often associated with violence can be divided into four categories:

1. sedatives or depressants acting upon the central nervous system: alcohol, barbiturates, and diazepam (Valium)
2. stimulants: cocaine, amphetamines, caffeine, and nicotine
3. hallucinogens: PCP, LSD, and marijuana
4. narcotics: heroin, morphine, Demerol, and Dilaudid.

Alcohol

"Unquestionably the drug most abused is alcohol."[38] There is almost no evil under the sun that at one time or another has not been attributed to the use and abuse of alcohol. Violent behavior is, of course, no exception. Alcohol has great potential for violence in all three stages of abuse. Even in the earliest stages of intoxication, violence-prone individuals may take even a slight loosening of controls as permission to commit violent acts. This use of alcohol in the service of violence is often a very conscious action, as in the Western movies where the bad guys drink in the saloon before leaving to kill the good rancher and ravish his beautiful daughter. The use of alcohol, in this case, is for intoxication to increase cortical disinhibition and facilitate a planned action; that is, it releases the individual from fear of retribution and reduces cortical control over the expression of the anger that presumably is inherent in such an act. Another type of violence may also occur in the intoxication phase. Self-directed violence, or suicide, occurs among alcoholics up to 80 times more often than among nonalcoholics.[31] This seems to be particularly true among older alcohol abusers, especially middle-aged males.

The association between wife abuse, child abuse, and alcohol abuse has already been noted here. Suffice it to say that such behaviors also seem to occur in association with the intoxication phase. It may be legitimate to conclude that much of the purposeful, goal-directed violence occurring in association with alcohol use may occur in this stage.

Another potential source of violence during the intoxication stage is the behavioral change known as pathological intoxication, or, as the *Diagnostical Manual of Mental Disorders* (Third Edition) (DSM III) now terms it, alcohol idiosyncratic intoxication. This term refers to an extreme change in behavior, usually involving violence, following the imbibing of a very moderate amount of alcohol. This behavioral change usually occurs in someone for whom the resultant aggressive behavior is quite out of character. The evidence for this condition is largely anecdotal, and Hollender[39] has presented evidence that it really may be simply a dissociative reaction, since attempts to produce it in the laboratory have been futile to date.

Violence in the withdrawal stage tends to occur when alcohol withdrawal really is becoming uncomfortable, usually about the third day of abstinence. Alcohol abusers may then become violent in their demands for alcohol or other drugs. They may assault the persons denying these drugs or may actively pursue obtaining them in some other fashion. Less purposeful violence in the withdrawal phase may occur if they begin to experience alcohol hallucinosis, at which time they may resort to violence to avoid fantasied anticipated injury.

Somewhat similar violence can be experienced in conjunction with the delusions, hallucinations, and agitations experienced in the course of delirium tremens (d.t.'s). This condition, now termed by DSM III alcohol withdrawal delirium,[35] occurs in less than 5 percent of alcoholic patients, but it is a great source of concern when it does.

Violence may occur in the residual phase of alcohol abuse in connection with dementia. Dementia usually is observed clinically in alcohol abusers who have consumed excessive amounts of alcohol over a period of years. Memory and judgment are impaired, and when they are severely impaired, violence is more likely.

Barbiturates

Barbiturates act as depressants on the central nervous system. They usually are classified according to the duration of their action.[38,40] The categories are short-, medium-, and long-lasting. Many barbiturate abusers come to prefer the short-acting variety, with secobarbital (Seconal) a commonly preferred type.

Because of their depressant effect, which can produce gradual drowsiness, barbiturates are frequently used for suicide attempts. However, on occasion, these drugs can have an excitatory effect, causing excitability and hyperactivity. This action seems more common when the sleep cycle is interrupted.

During this excitable stage, striking out and other forms of violence are possible. Violence may also occur during the withdrawal stage, when the individual is actively seeking drugs to stave off the rebound effect from the barbiturates.

Diazepam (Valium)

It is ironic that Valium should be considered a drug associated with the potential for violence, since so often it is used as a calming agent, especially in treating the alcoholic in withdrawal. Kissin, in reviewing the drugs used in treating the effects of the abuse of ethyl alcohol, concluded that "...on the basis of available evidence, diazepam would appear to be the safest drug for reducing agitation in acute alcohol intoxication."[41] Nevertheless, it is my clinical experience that Valium use can be associated with violent behavior. While there is growing concern about its use, it continues to be seen in health care settings as one of the more common of the misprescribed drugs. It seems to be particularly popular among alcoholics in the service of the denial of their addiction. Thus, alcoholics may proudly boast that they have stopped drinking for perhaps two years or more. Careful questioning, however, may then yield the information that the individual has accomplished this feat by ingesting heavy doses of Valium over this period and is now presenting with many of the addictive symptoms noted with alcohol dependency, including severe withdrawal symptoms. If anything, the withdrawal period for Valium is even more prolonged than that for alcohol, and may include irritability and oppositionalism, which sometimes set the stage for violent behavior in the health care setting.

Amphetamines

Amphetamines, or "speed," are stimulants that have frequently been associated with violent behavior.[42] These drugs are associated with violence in one of two ways. As a stimulant, they can cause euphoric feelings in the violence-prone individual. Other effects can include suspiciousness, great fluctuations in mood, feelings of grandiosity, extreme physical activity, and great irritability. The effects are greatly enhanced by injection of the drug, as opposed to oral ingestion. Behavior in active "speed freaks" is quite unpredictable; they may be overly reactive to relatively mild and minor stimulation from their environments.

Even more dangerous are the persons presenting in the health care setting with an amphetamine-induced paranoid psychosis, or amphetamine toxicosis. The observable symptoms are indistinguishable from cases of paranoid psychosis or acute paranoid schizophrenia. In psychological tests, these individuals appear to exhibit paranoid schizophrenia, but as the effects of the drug diminish over a long period of time, the results of such tests may return to more normal levels. While this condition may result from one extremely powerful dose, it is more likely to be the result of long-term injection of amphetamines.

Cocaine

Cocaine seems to have become a prestige drug in this decade. Its primary attraction to users seems to lie in its initial effect, that of exquisite euphoria, with pleasurable disinhibition, since it is a most powerful stimulant drug. With heavy use, it can generate extreme depression and result in a toxic psychosis. There is potential for violence in all these stages. The agitated, paranoid cocaine user has great potential for almost any type of violence and is extremely unpredictable. For more extensive coverage of cocaine abuse, see Spotts and Shantz.[43]

Lysergic Acid Diethylamide (LSD)

Siva Sankar notes that the use of LSD extends over what he terms the initial stages, the experience itself, the recovery stage, and the aftermath.[44] Violent behavior is possible in all these stages because of possible anxiety and hallucinatory experiences. The reported "flashback" experience of some users, even after a period of several years, makes it important for the health care worker to know about the presenting individual's past use of LSD.

Marijuana

Marijuana is, after alcohol, caffeine, and nicotine, one of the most widely used of drugs. It is best classified as a mild hallucinogen, but as Fort[45] points out, it has both sedative and stimulant properties. This biphasic property probably makes possible the finding by Simonds and Kashani,[37] on the one hand, that marijuana is highly correlated with violence against persons, and the discovery by Tinklenberg et al.[14] on the other hand, that the 293 male juvenile offenders in their study selected marijuana as the drug that, in the considerable experience of these users, had the most calming effect.

In the health setting context, marijuana use is not ordinarily a consideration in anticipating violent behavior. There are, however, two conditions experienced by marijuana users that may contribute to violence. One of these is disinhibition of cortical control over aggressive impulses. This loosening of learned controls over aggression is similar to that found in the use of other intoxicants. The other, usually seen in heavy users over a long period of time, seems to be a more toxic, residual condition that may take some time, even months, to dissipate. Brecher[46] presents the interesting hypothesis that violence under the influence of marijuana actually may be generated by the dissemination of horror stories about its effects.

Phencyclidine (PCP)

There is evidence[47] that PCP has great potential for engendering violent behavior in the user, especially during the intoxication phase. Hallucinatory behavior with intense agitation and accompanying violence is a common observation. The violence is frequently nonspecific and not particularly goal-directed. PCP abusers also often report incidents of violent behavior and loss of behavioral control during flashback experiences occurring even years after PCP use. Of course, many PCP users were not the most stable of personalities before using PCP, and there is a distinct possibility that such persons are merely exhibiting dissociative manifestations and psychotic behaviors that might have occurred without a history of PCP use.

In a study of 16 chronic PCP users, Fauman and Fauman[48] found that their subjects gave little or no history of violent behavior, except when under the influence of drugs, suggesting that the PCP was largely responsible for the aggression that they exhibited. These authors also noted that their subjects committed acts that can be divided into four types of violence: relatively goal-oriented violence, impulsive violence, violence that is unexpected and bizarrely goal-oriented, and violence associated with agitation of psychotic quality. Wright[49] confirmed Fauman and Fauman's observations about the relationship between PCP and violence.

Most of the evidence suggests that PCP-related violence occurs during active use of the drug. There is some controversy about the incidence of such violence as a residual result solely of chronic PCP abuse. For example, Khajawall et al. reviewed the incidence of aggression during a 16-month period on a PCP ward. They compared these results with those from a heroin ward for the same period. They found "a relatively low level of overt aggressive and impulsive behavior."[47] Although there are methodological difficulties with this study, it does suggest that the correlation between PCP and violence may not be as clear as is frequently assumed. No matter what the parameters of the relationship between PCP and violence may be, there seems little doubt in the minds of health practitioners that there is some very strong connection.

Diacetylmorphine (Heroin)

Heroin is the narcotic most often associated with violent behavior in this culture. As is implied by its chemical name, it is a derivative of morphine, the active principle of opium. Its potential for abuse and for increasing physical and psychological dependence is well known. It has a sedative effect, similar to alcohol and barbiturates. Heroin becomes associated with violence most often in the withdrawal stage, when attempts are made to secure relief from the withdrawal symptoms, usually by obtaining the money for more, or by obtaining other narcotics directly from the health care provider. The residual effects are usually more psychological than physiological.

Lithium

Lithium salts in different forms are most often used in the treatment of bipolar affective (manic-depressive) disorders. While they seem most effective for patients with clearly documented manic phases, they are also used for treatment of recurrent schizoaffective disorders and some types of depressive disorders. (For a discussion, consult Kline and Angst,[38] pp. 196-199.) When associated with violent behavior in health care settings, lithium either has been used improperly or has been mixed with drugs such as alcohol, marijuana, or prescribed medications. The clinical picture of the violent lithium misuser is frequently one of an individual with increasing irritability and confusion, with eventual striking out, at first verbally, then, if not properly managed, physically against either person or property, or both.

Just as building the lithium level to a proper therapeutic level in the body is a slow, gradual process requiring constant monitoring, so, too, is the progress of lithium abatement after a period of lithium misuse that has precipitated violent behavior. If the underlying condition is a schizophrenic process, improvement may be particularly difficult and prolonged, perhaps even taking months for restabilization.

Mixed Drugs

Perhaps the greatest potential for violence occurs when the aggressor is under the influence of a combination of drugs. A drug that by itself is ordinarily harmless actually may exacerbate the effect of another drug. Generally, this phenomenon occurs during the intoxication phase of abuse. A good example would be marijuana, which, especially in moderate doses, produces relatively little violent behavior, and is seen by many as having a calming effect. However, when used with alcohol, it may result in excitatory behavior that may then eventuate in violence. Alcohol is the great synergic potentiator with many drugs. A good example is the alcohol-barbiturate combination, a frequent grouping in inadvertent suicides. Heavy users of alcohol experience the biphasic results of alcohol. At first, the alcohol is a calming agent, but it also produces some degree of anxiety. As the person becomes more tolerant of the alcohol, sleep becomes more difficult. At that time, the person may resort to barbiturates to sleep. Unfortunately, the synergic effect of these two central nervous system-depressing drugs may be, and often has been, fatal.

Alcohol, in combination with amphetamines, can also produce violent behavior. This is more likely to occur when the person is acutely intoxicated; the amphetamines then act to increase the excitation.[41]

Violence may also be observed in heroin addicts who combine alcohol with heroin. However, even more frequently observed is violence associated with alcohol in the heroin addict enrolled in a methadone program. Alcohol addiction seems to be a frequent occurrence, because the person on methadone misses the high formerly obtained from heroin, but absent when methadone is substituted.

Another potentially violent combination is amphetamines and barbiturates. Persons who begin to try to regulate their sleep-wake cycles with this combination may become more and more irritable, hyperactive, impulsive, and paranoid. They may then become prone to overreact to even the mildest of provocations with great vehemence.

Chemicals, Violence, and Psychiatric Illnesses

For several years, there has been disagreement (as discussed by Kenneth Tardiff in his chapter) concerning whether violent behavior is more frequent among psychiatric patients than in the population at large.[50,51,52,53] There now seems to be a growing consensus that the earlier studies suggesting a lower incidence of violent behavior among those with psychiatric illness may not present a complete and current picture. The links between psychiatric illness and violence are examined in Tardiff's chapter in this volume on the psychiatric patient. Clinical experience would certainly seem to indicate such a link, particularly when the effects of chemical abuse are added to the picture. One problem with the chemical-abusing patient is that drug misuse tends to uncover and exacerbate other conditions. For example, individuals with an underlying schizophrenic thought disorder may be able to deal effectively with their sense of alienation, loneliness, and rejection by others on a day-to-day basis for long periods of time. However, even occasional use of alcohol, marijuana, amphetamines, or barbiturates may be sufficient to elicit acute excitation, hallucinatory behavior, delusional thought, extreme confusion, profound dejection, or other manifestations of active and incapacitating psychosis.

In such individuals, the residual effect can be devastating, with the manifested symptomatology persisting for months or even years afterward. Should the individuals deny the idea of a connection between the chemical ingestion and their deteriorated functioning, as is all too often the case, a pattern of alternating periods of lucidity and dementia can become a way of life. Gradually, the lucid periods may become briefer and the disturbed periods longer, until the respites no longer occur. Frequently, treatment staff fail to deal adequately with such individuals because they tend to present atypical clinical features. They may be received initially by legal authorities, sent to a clinic or hospital, and treated only as a chemical abuser, especially if alcohol is the precipitating agent. As the immediate physical effect of the chemical wanes, the continuing symptomatology encourages a referral to a psychiatric setting. There, the focus may be solely on treatment of the psychiatric disorder, and the original chemical use may be ignored. The treated individuals will deny the circular causality of the condition and will not call attention to anything that may interrupt the denial system, especially if it may also disrupt their receipt of psychotropic drugs or invite a referral to a chemical treatment program that will discourage the use of "crutches" for their illnesses. Sensitivity to such interactive effects between chemicals and either psychiatric illnesses or personality traits (for the less psychiatrically oriented) becomes a crucial requirement for the health care worker in dealing with cases of violence. Understanding the nature of the person can aid greatly in the anticipation of the violence, and an understanding of the possible underlying psychopathology can increase knowledge of the impetus toward violence. It would be ideal, of course, if the worker could know in advance the psychiatric condition of all presenting patients. This is not always possible, particularly in admissions areas. Nevertheless, presenting personality characteristics can be used to assess violent potential, provided that the worker has some basic understanding of the violence of psychopathology and of the drug characteristics already mentioned.

Violence can be understood and classified in many ways. It can be goal-directed or entirely random and purposeless. It can be directed against the self or against a particular person or object, or, it can be totally without direction. Most violence in health care settings, however, arises out of feelings of fear or anger, or sometimes both. How the worker handles violence may depend on that worker's assessment of the source of the violence. This assessment is greatly facilitated by first assessing the characteristics of the individual or patient.

The Paranoid Patient

These individuals will be hostile and suspicious, but also highly fearful. Under the influence of chemicals, they may become extremely unpredictable and must be approached with caution at all times. Even the most casual touch may be interpreted by such a person as a deadly assault. The paranoid's behavior is often goal-directed in a highly personalistic manner.

The Schizophrenic Patient

This patient may exhibit a range of emotions, but has high potential for violence when under the influence of chemicals. Violent behavior may be goal-directed, but highly personalistic. It may also be nonspecific, especially when the individual is confused, delusional, or hallucinatory. Chemicals are often used to blunt subjective feelings of discomfort or to gain acceptance in some referent group.

One of the more striking examples of this attempt at acceptance involves a thirty-nine-year-old man diagnosed and treated as a paranoid schizophrenic. After leaving the hospital in remission, he returned to a rather lonely existence. With only limited social skills, his one affiliative activity was standing on the streets and drinking alcohol with a peer group. To gain greater status in this group, he increased his alcohol consumption and occasionally injected battery acid into his arm. He sought admission to an alcohol treatment program and assaulted an admissions worker who attempted to direct him to a psychiatric unit.

The Sociopathic Patient

This type of patient, particularly in violent situations, is characterized by angry, impulsive, poorly considered actions. Part of the antisocial behavior may include drug abuse. Drugs also are used frequently as an outlet and release for angry feelings or to boost courage. The behavior is usually goal-directed.

The Demented Patient

The demented patient is typically confused, often disoriented in time, place, and person, and frequently has great gaps in memory. The causation may be an effect of the drug itself or of some type of organic brain syndrome. Violence is likely to be nonspecific.

The Manic Patient

The manic patient is likely to be quite euphoric, with rapid, accelerated speech and motor agitation. The mania may stem from the effects of such drugs as PCP, amphetamines, or cocaine. The source also may be an affective disorder, and the behavior may be due to misuse of lithium. Behavior may be difficult to predict, but it is likely to be purposeful.

The Depressed Patient

This patient will exhibit great sadness, possibly with motor retardation. Suicidal behavior is possible. However, some patients convert depression into anger, and outwardly directed violence is also possible. This is particularly true under the effects of a depressive drug such as alcohol.

The Demanding, Belligerent Patient

Aggressive, belligerent behavior on the part of any patient signals the potential for violence, particularly when drugs are either demanded or in use by the patient. The source of violence can be drug withdrawal, a characterological personality, severe psychopathology, or the effect of a chemical. The behavior is usually goal-directed and can rapidly escalate to a higher level of violence.

The Delirious Patient

The typical delirious patient is experiencing the effects of withdrawal from alcohol. This patient's violent behavior will usually be random and nondirected.

Assessing And Anticipating Violent Behavior In The Chemical Abuser

The best protection against the consequences of violent behavior for both the patient and the health care worker is the anticipation and defusing of violent actions. Several writers[32,33,54-57] have suggested strategies and protocols for the assessment of such behaviors. While an exhaustive review of such strategies will not be attempted here, it is possible to consider some of the more important elements involving the chemical abuser.

The particular health care setting is one important consideration. Violent incidents involving drug abusers are more likely to occur in emergency room settings, drug or alcohol treatment units, detoxification centers, and psychiatric wards. This is particularly true if the settings are open wards or long-term treatment facilities. General hospital wards that admit acute medical patients are also possible locations.

Time is an important consideration and one that interacts with the settings. The more obvious relationship is that between Saturday nights and the level of activity in emergency rooms, especially during the "party hours" on either side of midnight. Stokeman[53] mentions that patients in both general and forensic psychiatric hospitals are more likely to be violent immediately following admission to the hospital and during meals. The so-called sundown syndrome is well-known in geriatric hospitals, but the concept is probably valid for most hospital settings: violence often occurs on the evening shift, a time when staffing is usually rather low and when some inpatients may have had nefarious visitors or made surreptitious trips outside the ward.

The location of the health care setting can be a factor. Violence, and especially violence correlated with chemical abuse, is to be anticipated more in facilities in large, urban settings, where illicit drugs are more readily available than in smaller, more rural settings. Violent behavior also is more likely in units serving ghettos than those serving a more affluent clientele, for a variety of reasons, including class differences, staffing ratios, sheer patient volume, and the expectations of staff and patients. However, it is probable that no location is totally immune from this type of violence, including prison settings.

The treatment or personal history of the chemical abusing individual is also an important consideration. If persons have past histories of violent behavior, whether drug-related or not, they are much more likely to be risks for such behavior than are persons who have not previously resorted to such actions. A history of use of violence-related drugs or of psychiatric diagnosis observed in connection with violent behavior is also a warning signal to carefully assess the potential for present violent behaviors.

The presenting situation is also a prime consideration. An individual brought in by a police officer in handcuffs must be assessed very carefully, but an individual brought in by five or six officers must be evaluated even more carefully. A person who appears to be accompanied by a spouse with whom he or she is engaged in violent verbal interaction may well transfer angry feelings from the spouse to the health care worker with little or no encouragement, especially if the accompanying spouse tells the worker to "fix the patient." It might be added that the accompanying spouse may also displace angry feelings to the worker, and thus bears watching.

The physical appearance of the patient should also be considered. The disheveled, ill-kempt person with poor personal hygiene may well be violent. It should be remembered, however, that many very dangerous paranoid patients are extremely meticulous about their personal appearances, even during periods of prolonged violence.

Motoric behavior may be another warning to assess for violent potential. The individual who paces agitatedly, or who alternately approaches and then retreats from the staff member, may be gathering courage for an assault or may be struggling with unbearable, unacceptable, or uncontrollable violent impulses. The wild look of some paranoid or drug-related states is a well-known sign for caution.

I am acquainted with one individual who dramatically signals his assaultive intent with his eyes. He begins to exhibit an expanded sense of his personal space, which extends to include all activity within about eight feet of himself—just about the width of a hallway. These periods of threat arise after ingestion of small amounts of ethyl alcohol or shaving lotion. He begins to signal his feeling of being personally threatened either by totally avoiding eye contact or by staring intently at potential victims. At such times, it is most prudent to avoid eye contact and to increase physical distance from him. Another example is a patient whose violence is signaled by frequent trips to the water fountain. As his level of water intoxication builds, so does his irritability and potential for explosive behavior.

Other motoric clues may include speech characteristics. Persons agitated by use of amphetamines or those in manic states may exhibit great rapidity of speech. At the other end of the speech spectrum, the depressed patient will sometimes show either greatly accelerated or decelerated speech or movement. It is the dramatic change in speed of movement that may be a clue to a pending change in behavior, which may include a suicidal act.

The content of speech or writing may be important. The person who commits a violent act may talk or write about it, or even paint it, for some time before actually doing it. The person whose speech content is confused is reflecting confused thought, which can sometimes eventuate in confused and violent acts.

Staff Considerations

To this point, only the history and actions of the potentially violent individual have been presented. Less often discussed are actions and attitudes that may be just as important as those of patients: the characteristics of the health care workers. Just as the potential for violence in a setting can be assessed by carefully evaluating the patient, it is also important to assess the health care staff and their environments.

The process of properly assessing and anticipating violent behavior must include consideration of the health care staff and its patterning. In reviewing violent incidents occurring in health care settings, it is quite common to find points where a proper staff action or inaction might have defused a violent incident. Anticipating violence, therefore, must include an assessment of those elements in a situation that are resolvable by health care workers.

Most violent episodes, even those involving drugs, center around the emotions of fear and anger. If the staff member contributes to these emotions, for whatever reason, instead of allaying them, then the potential for a violent incident increases. Many conditions make it more likely that workers will contribute adversely, generally because of their own fears or frustrations, but sometimes out of ignorance; these conditions must be assessed.

In assessing the situation for violent potential, it is well to start with the quality and extent of communication, because so many human problems stem from poor communication. Poor or incomplete communication breeds a disturbed and insecure environment for patients or staff members, and an insecure situation enhances the chance of violence.

Health care settings are among the most stressful of working environments,[58] because the consequences of even small oversights can be so catastrophic in human terms. In such environments, small problems become greatly magnified. Minor disruptions in organization rapidly can become chaos.

There are many clues to use in detecting the presence of stressed staff members. One of the most important is the lack of a unifying health philosophy. If a staff group has no common purpose, no common language that is shared at all levels, frustrations will build between staff members and create uneasiness between staff and patients. Patients then feel more threatened and begin to test the structure; staff also then feel more threatened and fatigued. Some staff members may transfer their frustrations about their work conditions to patients. In this way, the stage is set for violent incidents. Drug usage becomes a volatile catalyst in such situations.

Another clue to stressed staff is the presence of such poor morale indicators as high staff turnover, high rates of absenteeism, and high numbers of on-the-job injuries. Such indicators are great predictors of violent potential, not only because they indicate staff dissatisfactions, but because of the disruption in unit routine that they inevitably generate. Also, gaps in staffing often create a sense of fright and apprehension, both for patients and staff.

Water-cooler conversations among the staff, often overheard by patients, may give clues to staff frustrations and dissatisfactions, as well as to problems in the organization. If the content of such conversations includes great anger for lack of support from the administration, then the organization has problems. Similarly, if the topics habitually suggest great problems in the personal lives of the staff, then job performance may suffer.

Other clues may be key events in the health setting, including pending inspections by accrediting agencies, construction or remodeling of the physical setting, actions by governing authorities, the level of patient population and rates of turnover, shortages of critical supplies and equipment, and loss of critical personnel or positions.

Finally, staff members sometimes take a number of adverse actions that can be instrumental in precipitating violence on the part of someone inclined toward violence, but who, to that point, has not received the stimulus to act out. Like it or not, in the final analysis, health care workers must deal with the fact that their actions frequently can determine the course of a violent event. Often, such actions are routine in everyday life, and would be so construed by the average person. However, in this totally different context, such actions may be redefined and reinterpreted by a less than rational person. Health care staffs should appreciate this possibility, and some examples may help them to do so.

Anger is frequently elicited in a patient by the worker who is overly officious in manner, who is quite brusque, who speaks in a steadily rising voice, who has a sharp tone, and who uses threats to gain compliance. If such a worker adds to this picture by pointing a finger, paranoid or hypersensitive patients may well interpret this action as a direct threat to their rather fragile sense of "manhood."

At the other extreme is the worker who mumbles and speaks hesitantly, in a tone so low as to be nearly inaudible to the patient. Patients may become quite threatened by such an individual and feel that the worker is trying to deceive or mislead them. If such a worker takes actions with the patient that the patient does not understand and that the worker does not explain, then distrust is multiplied.

Another mistake workers often make is to become so concerned with achieving compliance from the patient that they forget that they are dealing with someone who has a great deal of pathology. Such workers will often become quite insistent on fairly minor points in the face of strong opposition from the patient. An example would be the worker who insists that the patient be separated from someone on whom the patient is strongly dependent for emotional support during a highly stressful event, such as entering an emergency room. In such a case, the staff member may have to make a decision about whether to simply manage the patient or to engage that individual in a mutually shared treatment process.

Lecturing, criticizing, failing to listen, and failing to respect the patient as an individual with rights and dignity can also potentiate violence. In violence-prone situations, perhaps the crucial skill is to listen, not just to the patient, but to the illness or pathological condition.

As a further example, the paranoid patient frequently has a greatly expanded field of personal space. Intrusions into this space, especially rapid movements, can be highly threatening, as can unexpected and silent approaches from behind the patient. In addition, turning one's back on patients can be interpreted as rejection of their needs, which may invite retaliatory expressions of rage.

Keeping patients waiting for long periods when they are in acute emotional or physical distress is also dangerous. Also, it is foolhardy to leave potentially violent patients in isolation with limited freedom to move about; this increases feelings of fear and rage.

Finally, as a general rule, it is not wise to be alone in the presence of someone who has been seen as potentially violent, especially if that person is under the influence of drugs. This may allow the patient to focus too much violent emotion upon one person in the environment, and may make it difficult to summon aid in the event of violence.

Management of the Violent Chemical Abuser

The effective operation of any organizational unit requires proper management. This is especially true of units in which the structure can be tested by
violent behavior. Maximizing the effectiveness of such units secures the
survival of the unit, the patient, and the staff. The incidence of violence can
be reduced by careful managerial planning.

The first step in the establishment of a unit in which violent behavior can
be handled effectively is to develop clear statements of the function and
purpose of such a unit. A unifying philosophy for the unit is crucial; it should
be clearly articulated and congruent with the environment. Operation of the
unit should be administratively monitored for continued compliance with the
guidelines thus articulated; such monitoring is best accomplished in a
facilitative manner, not one that will prove disruptive to the actual operation
of the unit.

The next step is to select the personnel for the unit. The professional
credentials for the staffs will differ from setting to setting, depending on the
institutional structures and purposes. However, the selection of the personnel
for a unit where violence may occur is very important for the organization as
a whole. Too often, such units are staffed with individuals inadequate to
handle the violent patient. Instead, the emphasis should be on hiring
individuals outstanding for employment in such areas.

Personal characteristics desirable for the effective violence manager are the
same as those for any first-class health professional. Professional and
technical knowledge are to be assumed. This type of staff member needs to be
calm under pressure and have great flexibility, creativity, and resourcefulness.
Being able to listen to patients and to empathize objectively are very
necessary skills. Staff members also need to have assertiveness and self-
confidence without arrogance or undue aggressiveness to be able to function
in the context of a crisis team when required to do so. Organizational ability
and the competence to function in a unit are also requisites.

Once such personnel are in place, they must define for themselves how they
will function in the face of a violent situation. Lines of authority and
responsibility must be clearly delineated in such contexts, since there will be
no time to make such decisions during an incident. For such violent
confrontations, lines of authority will depend on the pertinent knowledge of
the individual staff members involved, rather than on the disciplines they
represent. The individuals with the most expertise in such matters, or those
with critical duties, whatever their specialties, are to be in lead roles, with
other personnel assisting as needed.

These authoritative personnel determine those operational procedures that
will ultimately simplify their tasks. One example is the scheduling of available

staff members. Staffing patterns need to take into account the data presented here that suggests that violent incidents are more likely at certain times or on certain occasions, for example, at meal times, in the evenings, or shortly after admission.

Decisions also must be made about unit policies on such issues as visitors to the unit, visiting hours, pass inspections of patient areas, and any other topics of interest to ward management. Clarity in such policies and consistency in their application will aid greatly in forestalling potential conflicts about such issues.

Attention must be directed to the physical characteristics of the unit. Location of nursing stations or offices and patient areas should be planned for maximum safety. In inpatient units, the staff needs clear views of potential conflict spots. In emergency rooms, the staff must be able to encounter patients in areas where they can be contained, if necessary, but where the staff members will not be entrapped. There needs to be an absolute minimum of loose equipment that could be employed as weapons. Furniture should not lend itself to use as weapons. Metal or wooden charts are to be in secure places. Oxygen bottles are to be mounted on walls, not loose or free-standing, and there should be no unattended litters or wheelchairs.

The interior decor needs to be more than an afterthought. In areas where acute patients will be received, such as emergency or admission areas, it is well to keep distractions to a minimum. Soothing colors are helpful, because excessive stimulation may aggravate some persons in acute drug states. On the other hand, where patients may reside for long periods, and where depressive states may predominate, somewhat livelier, though not garish, colors may be desired.

Care should also be exercised in the establishment of a recording system. Record-keeping can be both a curse and a blessing for the health care facility, especially as it pertains to the emergent situation. An adequate record of violent incidents is essential to avoid legal entanglements, to facilitate staff communications in the interest of good patient treatment, and to maintain accreditation standards. A quick-reference card system may be helpful in treating frequently readmitted patients. Color flagging charts of patients with past histories of violent behavior may help personnel by warning them to maintain extra vigilance around those persons.

The curse of record-keeping is that it can become tremendously time-consuming for the staff. It can even contribute to the genesis of violence when it becomes so much a focus of staff activity that proper monitoring of patient behavior suffers. All too often, there is an apparent assumption by health care managers that the staff can always be given more paper work—special studies, reports, new monitoring forms—with no detriment in terms of patient care. This is almost never a valid assumption. The addition of one extra minute of paper work, of one extra special procedure, reduces staff interaction with the potentially violent person by one minute—or more, if one considers the time required to replace forms when supplies run low and that staff member must be dispatched for a new batch. Allocation of time to orient new staff to the paper work must also be considered.

The natural inclination of the clinicians who are "in the trenches" is to attempt to reject out of hand paper work that they believe interferes with patient care. There is sometimes some justification for this view, particularly if the paper work requirement is not carefully planned, reviewed, and utilized in the justifiable interest of quality patient care.

An example of such paper work is reviews of violent incidents in hospitals. Most psychiatric hospitals, in adherence to the standards required for accreditation by the Joint Commission for the Accreditation of Hospitals (JCAH), require that incidence reports be completed by personnel when violent incidents occur, and that these reports be compiled and reviewed by hospital administration. In cases of violent incidents, nursing personnel are required to fill out the details of the incidents on forms designed for that purpose. The forms are then reviewed by administrative committees appointed for that purpose. Often, the review results are not made known to the line staff, except for an occasional commendation to an individual staff member who handled a particular incident in exemplary fashion, or for an equally occasional reprimand to a staff member who erred.

Employing such reports in this manner frequently produces the attitude on the part of line staff that the incident report is only in that baneful category of punitive and unnecessary paper work, done only for the convenience of a distant body that does not understand what goes on at the firing line. The implications for labor-management relationships, morale, and ultimate patient care are obvious.

Contrast the preceding administrative approach with one in which such reports are used in an atmosphere of mutual problem solving as one more helpful tool for meeting clearly stated goals and for continuing staff development, not only for the purpose of seemingly arbitrary reward and punishment. Properly used, these reports become a valuable tool for operational feedback, aiding in self-correction of operational procedures by staff members. This approach can also generate in the staff a sense of confidence and participation in management.

Davidson et al.[59] report an example of the use of clearly defined policies and feedback to produce positive change in a large center for the mentally retarded. The purpose of the administration was to reduce the use of psychotropic drugs, restraints, and seclusion with residents. To accomplish this goal, behavioral data on the use of such measures was collected. The administrator of the facility clearly defined the goal of reducing the use of such procedures. The data was then reviewed and made available at a variety of levels, from the interdisciplinary teams on each unit to the state department of mental health. The result of these measures was a significant reduction in the use of all of the three restrictive treatment procedures.

Unit planners should also direct their attention to the development of a training plan for the education of the individual staff members. Such training is to be both general—that is, applicable to all the unit staff and operation of the unit—and specific, or applicable to individual members for special training needs. Opportunity should be available for staff members to receive the benefit of training away from the home institution. Such well-planned training ensures fresh ideas and aids in reducing staff burnout.

The unit needs appropriate support services to augment the efforts of the line staff. Sufficient clerical support spares the need for the clinical staff to perform clerical duties. Laboratory test results should be timely; especially in cases of drug use, lab results that are available in three days to a week are essentially useless for good clinical management, although they may meet a need for ensuring legal protection. Standby security personnel should also be planned for in most institutional settings.

Finally, personnel must determine for themselves their day-to-day operational philosophies and techniques as they pertain to violent individuals within the mandate from their general institutional setting. In this regard, there are many schools of thought on the management of the violent individual, ranging from what might be termed the "superior firepower" school of surrounding and subduing the violent individual, to the "lone therapist" approach by which only one person tries to deal with the violent individual. All of these schools have their advocates. None can be guaranteed to work in all situations because of the complexities involved. Nevertheless, there are some general guidelines.

As an example, Stine et al.[34] have noted that such approaches as isolating the patients or touching them during a violent episode can be ineffective. They also deplore as ineffective an atmosphere of suspicion, distrust, or hostility, as well as one in which the staff is very physically or emotionally distant from the individual. Conversely, they cite role modeling, patient awareness, positive reinforcement, and the opportunity for the individual to express anger as important for the effective management of violence.

On a practical level, many violent episodes seem to build in a sequence from mild anger to explosiveness. Management techniques also can be viewed in sequence, although the point at which violence management begins in the sequence is usually dependent on the stage at which the violent individual is encountered:

Stage 1. *Educative.* Here, workers can attempt to discuss with the patients what is happening and why. Reassurance is given. Reasoning is attempted.
Stage 2. *Avoidance.* If possible, confrontation is avoided. If the individuals can cool down on their own, with a minimum of monitoring, they are allowed to do so.
Stage 3. *Appeasement.* This may or may not be possible. If the individuals have weapons and demand available drugs, accommodation may be the wisest course. If the demands are really simple or reasonable, although made in a belligerent and bellicose fashion, it may be better to grant the demands and worry about the lessons to be learned later.
Stage 4. *Deflection.* If the violence is related to topics that can be shifted, this should be done.
Stage 5. *Time out.* The individuals may be persuaded to retire to a space set aside for them to be alone and think things over, with reduced stimulation.
Stage 6. *Show of force.* It may be necessary to forcibly show patients to a timeout room, generally using at least enough workers to subdue each of the patients' extremities, plus personnel to open doors or to add restraints if that becomes necessary.
Stage 7. *Seclusion.* The patients may have to be locked in timeout rooms.
Stage 8. *Restraint.* The patients may have to be immobilized by mechanical restraints to prevent injury to themselves or others.
Stage 9. *Sedation.* The patients may have to be totally or partially sedated to prevent violence. This step can be especially risky and may have to be avoided if possible with persons who have ingested unknown drugs. Mild sedation, of course, may be introduced earlier in the sequence if other measures seem to offer little hope or need supplementation.

NOTES

1. L. W. Gerson, "Alcohol-related Acts of Violence: Who Was Drinking and Where the Acts Occurred," *Journal Studies on Alcohol* 39 (1978): 1294-6.

2. L. W. Gerson and D. A. Preston, "Alcohol Consumption and the Incidence of Violent Crime," *Journal Studies on Alcohol* 40 (1979): 307-312.

3. H. J. Steadman, "A Situational Approach to Violence," *International Journal of Law and Psychiatry* 5 (1982): 7-86.

4. A. R. Nicol, J. C. Gunn, and J. Gristwood, "The Relationship of Alcoholism to Violent Behavior Resulting in Long-term Imprisonment," *British Journal of Psychiatry* 123 (1973): 47-51.

5. D. Mayfield, "Alcoholism, Alcohol Intoxication and Assaultive Behavior," *Diseases of the Nervous System* 37 (1976): 288-291.

6. R. M. Viken, "Family Violence: Aids to Recognition," *Postgraduate Medicine* 71 (1982): 115-122.

7. J. A. Byles, "Violence, Alcohol Problems and Other Problems in Disintegrating Families," *Journal Studies on Alcohol* 39 (1978): 551-554.

8. T. C. Fleming, "Violence: The Role of Chemical Agents," *Postgraduate Medicine* 69 (1981): 27-8, 30.

9. R. M. Sarles, "Child abuse," in *Rage, Hate, Assault and Other Forms of Violence*, eds. D. J. Madden and J. R. Lion (New York: Spectrum, 1976), pp. 1-16.

10. K. C. Meiselman, *Incest* (San Francisco: Jossey-Bass, 1978).

11. R. E. Hemphill and Wendy Fisher, "Drugs, Alcohol and Violence in 604 Male Offenders Referred for Inpatient Psychiatric Assessment," *South African Medical Journal* 57 (1980): 243-247.

12. J. R. Tinklenberg et al., "Drug Involvement in Criminal Assaults by Adolescents," *Archives of General Psychiatry* 30 (1974): 685-689.

13. J. R. Tinklenberg and K. M. Woodrow, "Drug Use Among Youthful Assaultive and Sexual Offenders," in *Aggression*, ed. S. H. Frazier (Baltimore: Williams and Wilkins, 1974), pp. 209-224.

14. J. R. Tinklenberg et al., "Drugs and Criminal Assaults by Adolescents: A Replication Study," *Journal of Psychoactive Drugs* 13 (1981): 277-287.

15. K. Andersen, "Private violence," *Time*, September 5, 1983, pp. 18-19.

16. S. F. Bauer and L. Balter, "Emergency Psychiatric Patients in a Municipal Hospital: Demographic, Clinical and Dispositional Characteristics," *Psychiatric Quarterly* 45 (1971): 382-393.

17. D. Q. Hagen, J. Mikolachzak, and R. Wright, "Aggression in Psychiatric Patients," *Comprehensive Psychiatry* 13 (1972): 481-487.

18. J. M. Lagos, K. Perlmutter, and H. Saexinger, "Fear of the Mentally Ill: Empirical Support for the Common Man's Response," *American Journal of Psychiatry* 134 (1979): 1134-1139.

19. S. Marten, R. A. Munoz, and K. A. Gentry, "Belligerence: Its Frequency and Correlates in a Psychiatric Emergency Room Population," *Comprehensive Psychiatry* 13 (1972): 241-249

20. A. E. Skodol and T. B. Karasu, "Emergency Psychiatry and the Assaultive Patient," *American Journal of Psychiatry* 135 (1978), pp. 202-205.

21. M. Suh and R. Carlson, "A Socio-psychiatric Profile of Emergency Room Patients," *Canadian Journal of Psychiatry* 24 (1979): 219-223.

22. K. Tardiff and A. Sweillam, "Assault, Suicide and Mental Illness," *Archives of General Psychiatry* 37 (1980): 164-169.

23. R. M. Whitman, B. V. Armao, and O. B. Dent, "Assault of the Therapist," *American Journal of Psychiatry* 133 (1976): 426-429.

24. D. J. Madden, J. R. Lion, and M. W. Penna, "Assaults on Psychiatrists by Patients," *American Journal of Psychiatry* 133 (1976): 422-425.

25. G. Bach-Y-Rita, J. R. Lion, and C. E. Climent, "Episodic Dyscontrol: A Study of 130 Violent Patients," *American Journal of Psychiatry* 127 (1971): 1473-1478.

26. G. Bach-Y-Rita and A. Veno, "Habitual Violence: A Profile of 62 Men," *American Journal of Psychiatry* 134 (1974): 1015-1017.

27. J. R. Lion, G. Bach-Y-Rita, and F. R. Ervin, "Violent Patients in the Emergency Room," *American Journal of Psychiatry* 125 (1969): 1706-1711.

28. K. J. Tardiff, "A Survey of Psychiatrists in Boston and Their Work with Violent Patients," *American Journal of Psychiatry* 131 (1974): 1008-1011.

29. H. N. Ochitill and M. Krieger, "Violent Behavior Among Hospitalized Medical and Surgical Patients," *Southern Medical Journal* 75 (1982): 151-155.

30. American Psychiatric Association, *Clinical Aspects of the Violent Individual* (Washington, D.C.: American Psychiatric Association, 1974).

31. D. H. Marjot, "Alcohol, Aggression and Violence," *The Practitioner* 226 (1982): 287-294.

32. J. H. Atkinson, Jr., "Managing the Violent Patient in the General Hospital," *Postgraduate Medicine* 71 (1982): 193-201.

33. R. T. Rada, "The Violent Patient: Rapid Assessment and Management," *Psychosomatics* 22 (1981): 101-109.

34. Linda J. Stine, S. W. Patrick, and J. Molina, "What is the Role of Violence in the Therapeutic Community?" *International Journal of Addictions* 17 (1982): 377-392.

35. American Psychiatric Association, *Diagnostic and Statistical Manual of Mental Disorders*, 3rd ed. (Washington, D.C.: American Psychiatric Association, 1980).

36. National Commission on Marijuana and Drug Abuse, *Drug Use in America: Problem in Perspective* (Washington, D.C.: United States Government Printing Office, 1973).

37. J. F. Simonds and J. Kashani, "Specific Drug Use and Violence in Delinquent Boys," *American Journal of Drug and Alcohol Abuse* 7 (1980): 305-322.

38. N. Kline and J. Angst, *Psychiatric Syndromes and Drug Treatment* (New York: Jason Aronson, 1979).

39. M. H. Hollender, "Pathological Intoxication—Is There Such an Entity?" *Journal of Clinical Psychiatry* 40 (1979): 424-426.

40. National Clearinghouse for Drug Abuse Information, *CNS Depressants* (Rockville, Md: National Institute on Drug Abuse, 1974).

41. B. Kissin, "Interactions of Ethyl Alcohol and Other Drugs," in *The Biology of Alcoholism*, vol. 3, *Clinical Pathology*, eds. B. Kissin and H. Begleiter (New York: Plenum Press, 1974), pp. 109-161.

42. E. H. Ellinwood, Jr., "Amphetamine Psychosis: Individuals, Settings, and Sequences," in *Current Concepts of Amphetamine Abuse*, eds. E. H. Ellinwood and S. Cohen (Rockville, Md: National Institute of Mental Health, 1972), pp. 143-157.

43. J. V. Spotts and F. C. Shontz, *Cocaine Users: A Representative Case Approach* (New York: The Free Press, 1980).

44. D. V. Siva Sankar, *LSD—A Total Study* (Westbury, N.Y.: PJD Publications, 1975).

45. J. Fort, "LSD and the Mind-altering Drug (M.A.D.) World," in *The Problems and Prospects of LSD*, ed. J. T. Ungerleider (Springfield, Ill.: Charles C Thomas, 1968), pp. 3-21.

46. E. M. Brecher, ed., *Licit and Illicit Drugs: The Consumers Union Report on Narcotics, Stimulants, Depressants, Inhalants, Hallucinogens, and Marijuana—Including Caffeine, Nicotine, and Alcohol* (Boston: Little, Brown and Company, 1972).

47. A. M. Khajawall, T. B. Erickson, and G. M. Simpson, "Chronic Phencyclidine Abuse and Physical Assault," *American Journal of Psychiatry* 139 (1982): 1604-1606.

48. M. A. Fauman and B. J. Fauman, "Violence Associated with Phencyclidine Abuse," *American Journal of Psychiatry* 136 (1979): 1584-1586.

49. H. H. Wright, "Violence and PCP Abuse," *American Journal of Psychiatry* 137 (1980): 752-753.

50. D. J. Mulvihill and M. M. Tumin, *Crimes of Violence*, vol. 12, *Staff Report to the National Commission on the Causes and Prevention of Violence* (Washington, D. C.: U. S. Government Printing Office, 1969).

51. A. Zitrin et al., "Crime and Violence Among Mental Patients," *American Journal of Psychiatry* 133 (1976): 142-149.

52. J. M. Giovannoni and L. Gurel, "Socially Disruptive Behavior of Ex-mental Patients," *Archives of General Psychiatry* 17 (1967): 146-153.

53. C. L. J. Stokeman, "Q & A: Violence Among Hospitalized Mental Patients," *Hospital and Community Psychiatry* 33 (1982): 986.

54. C. K. Maynard and K. K. Chitty, "Dealing with Anger: Guidelines for Nursing Intervention," *Journal of Psychiatric Nursing and Mental Health Services,* June, 1979, pp. 36-41.

55. F. S. Tennant, Jr., "Physician Extender Protocols for Urgent Situations in Drug and Alcohol Clinics," *Journal of Psychedelic Drugs* 11 (1979): 211-215.

56. J. P. Tupin, "The Violent Patient: A Strategy for Management and Diagnosis," *Hospital and Community Psychiatry* 34 (1983): 37-40.

57. L. S. Lehmann et al., "Training Personnel in the Prevention and Management of Violent Behavior," *Hospital and Community Psychiatry* 34 (1983): 40-43.

58. G. L. Calhoun, "Hospitals Are High-stress Employers," *Hospitals* 54 (1980): 171-175.

59. N. A. Davidson, M. J. Hemingway, and T. Wysocki, "Reducing the Use of Restrictive Procedures in a Residential Facility," *Hospital and Community Psychiatry* 35 (1984): 164-167.

Chapter 8

The Men in Blue Pair Up with the People in White

Emily Friedman

Every hospital, no matter what its size or location, will sooner or later be visited by a police officer; it's a fact of hospital life. But the nature of the police presence in hospitals and the attitudes of police officers and hospital staff members can vary enormously. In New York City, police can be found, along with municipal judges, participating in the bedside arraignments of hospitalized prisoners. In Albuquerque, competition between police and sheriffs makes life even tougher for emergency department staffs. In Denver, the sheriffs who serve one hospital don't have to walk very far to get to their station house—it's in the hospital. In Oakland, CA, nurses ride along with police officers in squad cars to learn more about police procedures.

HANDCUFFS AND FISTICUFFS

The interaction between police officers and hospital employees can be anything from close and pleasant to distant and hostile; it can be formal or informal, structured or loose, effortless or painful. Its nature depends on what the hospital, the police department, and, most important, the individual officers and hospital staff members do to increase (or decrease) mutual understanding, define roles, and promote cooperation.

The size and location of the hospital and the police or sheriff's department are also contributing factors. For the small rural hospital, for instance, working with police is often not all that complicated. In Sundance, WY (population 800), the staff at Crook County Memorial Hospital and the local police officers are all neighbors, and their interactions normally go quite

---

Reprinted, with permission, from HOSPITALS, published by the American Hospital Association, copyright November 16, 1978, Vol. 52, No. 22.

smoothly. Dean Danielson, the hospital's former administrator, reports that "They all know each other. This is a ranching area, and there are cowboys who get drunk and hurt each other or themselves, but they do know that this is their community hospital, and they tend to mellow pretty well by the time they are brought here. They know that busting up the hospital would not be a very popular thing to do." If there is a disturbance, the police arrive quickly and handle it. In turn, when police bring in a prisoner who needs medical care, hospital personnel respond as quickly as possible.

At the other end of the spectrum is the damage that can be done when police officers and hospital staff members are *not* familiar with each other or with the procedures that are supposed to be followed in the hospital. On February 21, 1978, Hilda Sanabria, R.N., an emergency department (ED) nurse on the night shift at North Central Bronx Hospital, New York City, found herself handcuffed and arrested after a massive misunderstanding occurred between her and several police officers over the care of a handcuffed prisoner. Ms. Sanabria has asserted that the prisoner, who was bleeding when he arrived at the hospital, was being physically abused by the officers who had brought him in; the police assert that they were using reasonable force to quiet a violent prisoner who had already injured two policemen.

What actually happened is still in doubt, but the police officers, believing that Ms. Sanabria was interfering with their performance of their duties, arrested and handcuffed her and took her to the precinct house, where she received a summons and was released. She has filed suit against the city, the police department, and the two officers involved. She also filed a complaint with the New York City Police Department's Civilian Complaint Review Board (CCRB), which upheld the police officers.

The immediate conclusion one might draw is that the incident was not only bizarre, but unique—and that's not far from the truth. William T. Johnson, executive director of the CCRB, reports that of 3,500 complaints about police officers filed in the city each year, not more than 20 concern hospital-based incidents. Of these, many are complaints about police treatment of prisoners that are filed by hospital staff members. Others are clear-cut violations, including one recent incident when an off-duty police officer assaulted the driver of an ambulance after the officer's car had collided with it; the officer was arrested. "But these incidents are not frequent at all," Johnson reports.

A QUESTION OF DISCRETION

As it turns out, the Sanabria incident had at least one positive result: The local precinct and the hospital immediately started to work together to see that such an event would not happen again. Although the police involved in the case were not familiar with the hospital's ED staff—which, in fact, may have been one of the sources of the problem—it was obvious that better communications were needed even among the officers and ED staff who knew each other.

According to Harold Fingeret, executive director of North Central Bronx Hospital, the police made some immediate changes in procedure. Precincts were notified that under no circumstances were their officers to arrest an on-duty hospital employee unless he or she was committing a serious crime. If an arrest is necessary, the officer must consult his superior before making the arrest. In addition, the person being arrested can request that the borough police commander (who can be reached at any time, day or night) be consulted before the arrest is made.

Two encounter groups were held for ED staff and local police, with each group trying to explain its role in prisoner care and custody to the other. "Many things surfaced," Fingeret reports. "It allowed both sides to ventilate feelings. From these sessions came the idea of having additional meetings. . . . What essentially came out of it was a better understanding of each other's roles. The police came to understand that once they brought the person to the hospital, he really became a patient. . . . The initial effect of the incident on the staff was negative, but as a result of the discussions with the police, each side became more aware of the other's work. Also, checks were set up to avoid such a thing happening again. And we established ongoing communications with the police, which had been spotty previously."

One of the issues discussed during the meetings was the tricky question of when a patient must remain in handcuffs and when he can be freed from them. This is a question that comes up repeatedly in many hospitals. Johnson of the CCRB observes, "It's always a question of discretion. All hell can break loose once you *do* take them off." Fingeret believes that although the decision to remove cuffs rests with the police officer, he can and should listen to the advice of the hospital staff. The reverse is also true. Fingeret reports that one of the points made by officers in the encounter group meetings was that policemen have a "street sense" about potential violence on the part of hospitalized prisoners, and that this sense is more acute than a clinician's is. "If the police know that it took four cops to get the cuffs onto the prisoner, they are well-advised to be cautious about removing them. They don't want anyone getting hurt—*including themselves.* They are, after all, the people most likely to be injured by a violent prisoner," Fingeret says.

The question of when handcuffs stay on or come off usually is fairly clear-cut, with the police holding the ultimate authority; the problems that arise tend to be the product of misunderstandings on the part of hospital staff, or failure by officers to explain the necessity for keeping a patient handcuffed. Ed Stoltzenberg, associate executive director of Bellevue Hospital Center in New York City, reports that under Bellevue's procedures, "If cuffs must come off during an examination, a police officer will be present in the room. But our staff members are aware of the fact that handcuffs are necessary protection and are not cruel and unusual punishment."

A COLLISION OF RIGHTS

There are usually legal restrictions concerning the use of handcuffs, and specific handcuff policies are therefore commonplace in hospitals. Much more difficult are the myriad problems that can come up in which the law is fuzzy or contradictory, leaving hospital staff members and police to grope for a solution as best they can.

One common problem is that the very act of caring for a patient as speedily as possible can interfere with police needs, especially in the case of evidence. "Technically trained clinical staff can't be expected to think like law enforcement officers," in the opinion of Ben McGlaughlin, administrator of Auburn (CA) Faith Community Hospital.

Police report that it's a constant struggle to save evidence from the well-meaning hands of health care practitioners. Physicians at Bellevue, for example, were lax about marking bullets removed from patients, an oversight that in more than one instance spoiled the case against the assailant. The officers at the local precinct invited hospital staff members to headquarters and gave them a basic course in ballistics, including the marking of bullets.

At Providence Hospital in Oakland, CA, police requests led to the inclusion of information on basic police techniques in orientation for ED personnel. Among the most important requests was for patients' clothing to be preserved in one piece, as cutting through a bullet hole can ruin its potential role as a piece of evidence. Still, some problems defy easy solutions. Gerald Gordon, M.D., associate director of the emergency department at Denver General Hospital, has not been able to find an acceptable procedure for saving evidence of crimes that are discovered long after the patient is first admitted. The classic problematic case, he reports, occurs when a person comes in by ambulance as an emergency case, is treated, and then dies. A postmortem is performed, clothing and other artifacts are disposed of, and two days later the police find that the person was involved in a crime and that the corpse, the clothing, and other attendant items—which by then have been altered or destroyed—are key evidence. "It's a tough problem," Gordon says.

Another set of headaches stems from questions of patients' rights and confidentiality. One of the more unsettling laws that binds Bellevue employees (and those of all New York hospitals) is the provision that if a patient comes in for examination and is found to be carrying contraband (unregistered guns, drugs, or similar items), the hospital may confiscate the contraband but *may not* notify the police—it would be illegal to do so.

Therefore, staff members are unable to warn police about a potentially dangerous person, even though they may be in possession of evidence substantiating their fears. At Providence Hospital in Oakland, nurses can legally inform police in such situations, and they often do; they are not, however, required to report such information.

In terms of patients' medical records, the laws tend to be strict, and, by and large, police and detectives are not allowed access to them. This restriction leaves many hospital employees in the position of refusing access to irritated detectives who demand to see records, but the law will back up the hospital staff in most cases. A related matter is the desire on the part of police to photograph patients. Bernalillo County Medical Center in Albuquerque sought a legal opinion after a patient refused to allow himself to be photographed by police, and the police took pictures anyway. Legal research finally produced the opinion that the hospital had a right to refuse to allow patients to be photographed, because the patient had a clear right not to be photographed; the hospital, in giving consent for photographs, would be improperly assuming a "guardian" role that it did not have any legal basis for assuming.

CHECKING GUNS AT THE DOOR

In many cases, extremely difficult situations have been solved by careful development and use of protocols. For example, Bellevue is the only city hospital in New York that can admit prisoners who have not been arraigned. Once the patient has been assigned to a bed, a judge will come to the hospital and arraign him. These "bedside arraignments," which are unique to Bellevue, are never performed in the view of other patients; if the prison ward is full, the arraignment is held in a private room, a day room, or some other isolated place where the privacy of the prisoner—not to mention the mental and physical security of nonprisoner patients—is protected.

Psychiatric units also have developed highly sophisticated procedures to deal with the comings and goings of police. Under New York City law, a police officer may not surrender his weapon to anyone other than a superior officer; however, an armed police officer in a locked psychiatric ward is asking for trouble. Therefore, at Bellevue and other hospitals, the officer unloads his gun and leaves the bullets outside the ward. Even more sophisticated is the procedure at Denver General, where the officer unloads his gun, locks the bullets in one place, leaves the unloaded gun in a locked room, and then enters the ward. The reasoning behind the double-safety procedure is that even if a patient were able to break into the weapons room and obtain a weapon, the bullets for it would be nowhere around.

Psychiatric cases get more complicated outside the hospital in Denver. A "mental health hold"—an order that a patient be admitted for psychiatric reasons—can only be ordered by a police officer or a physician. Paramedics from Denver General cannot order a mental health hold, and they have reported being uneasy on some occasions when a police officer decides not to order a hold at the scene of a crime, when, in the paramedics' opinions, the patient presents a threat to the community. Equally unsettling to them is the situation when a police officer, usually after a traffic accident, allows a first-time offender to "get a break" and lets him go home. If that person has suffered a closed-head injury or an undetected trauma and later develops complications or dies, criticism is directed at the hospital and the ambulance crew for not bringing the patient in.

Lastly, there are the strange situations in which procedures must be made up as the hospital and the police go along. Ira Clark, executive director of Kings County Hospital Center in Brooklyn, vividly remembers the day that David Berkowitz, the accused "Son of Sam" murderer, was brought to the hospital for observation. The problems that occurred were not what might have been expected; the police were meticulously proper in their treatment of Berkowitz, and the hospital staff treated him like any other prisoner. The problem, Clark reports, was the near mob scene outside the hospital. "At the time of the arrest, because of the emotionalism and all the media attention, most of the police work that was needed was for outside security—perimeter security, plainclothes officers on the grounds and in the crowds outside the hospital, and so forth—while Berkowitz was being brought in. Once he was inside, penal officers took over in our prison unit, and there were no problems whatsover."

At Bellevue Hospital, it was discovered earlier this year that hospital employees were involved in loan sharking and drug dealing, a situation that is, unfortunately, common in large urban hospitals. The hospital staff did intelligence gathering and obtained some evidence, therefore providing the police with enough information to spark an undercover investigation. The investigation, which took a very short time, produced 10 major arrests. Stoltzenberg praises former Bellevue executive director Bernard M. Weinstein for confronting the situation publicly; hiding such information from the police, Stoltzenberg believes, would have been destructive for both the hospital and its employees.

Common sense is often the best protocol. Ralph Alvarado, deputy director of Lincoln Hospital in the Bronx, reports that at one New York City hospital (not Lincoln), a patient in the ED was found to be carrying a gun, for which he had a permit. Hospital personnel, who were uneasy about the patient, notified the hospital security force, and they, in turn, notified the police. The police, seeing that the patient had a permit, could not really do anything, although the hospital staff remained upset about the presence of the weapon in the hospital. The problem was solved when the administrator of the hospital simply asked the patient if he would relinquish the gun while he was being treated. That patient was quite willing to do so, and tensions were relieved all around.

"NOTHING BUT BLUE AND BLACK"

Another question that arises is whether it is preferable for police to be highly visible or to maintain a low profile when they are in hospitals. At St. Mary of Nazareth Hospital, Chicago, the administration believes that there is less chance of agitating emergency patients or staff if police officers are not highly visible; the hospital has therefore set up a "police room" next to its security station, where a table, chairs, a telephone, and a coffee machine are available to officers who are writing reports, waiting for a prisoner, or contacting precinct headquarters.

At other hospitals, different approaches are taken. At Kings County Hospital, Clark reports, "The police are so commonplace here that no one would be surprised to see them in the hospital. They're almost like the woodwork. That's good—I like the fact that the men in a radio car will come to the emergency department on a cold night for coffee." Likewise, the administration at Bellevue encourages policemen who are waiting at the hospital to "be seen" in the ED. "Bellevue likes to have uniformed police in full view," Stoltzenberg reports. "It adds an extra measure of security, and in an emergency department, that can make a great difference. You get a free addition to your security force for a while."

Sometimes space limitations can cause problems. Cheryl Scott, assistant administrator at Bernalillo County Medical Center, reports that the hospital's ED is so small that when police, sheriffs, and University of New Mexico policemen end up there in large numbers, the result is a huge traffic jam. Referring to the various uniforms milling around in a small, crowded place, Scott laments that sometimes "there's nothing but blue and black out there. We enjoy having them here; it's just that we have so little room." Such "police traffic jams" are normally easily dispersed. When one developed at Bellevue following the Wall Street ice-cream truck explosion earlier this year, the physician in charge of the ED asked all police to leave except for five officers; compliance was immediate.

Visibility also helps eliminate any chance that police actions will be misunderstood, especially in the delicate area of race relations. Clark observes, "Public-general hospitals in urban areas tend to be the refuge of minorities and the underclass, and these are not the groups that police tend to be most comfortable with. So police are not likely to overreact to provocation in the hospital setting; they know they are being watched by the staff and the patients, and therefore they are likely to behave differently than they will in a squad car or at the station." However, Clark adds, "prisoners know this and can take advantage of it." Scott adds that in Albuquerque, white police officers—and white citizens—are in the minority, and thus the "Anglo" officers take special care to be racially sensitive in the hospital setting and elsewhere.

A BOND OF UNDERSTANDING

At large hospitals, one way to eliminate friction between the hospital and the police is to have police assigned to the hospital. At one time, each New York City municipal hospital had a police officer assigned to it. City budget problems have ended the program at most hospitals, but at Bellevue, Officer Joe Butler's "beat" is serving as the liaison between the police department and the hospital. He recalls an era when the waiting time for officers whose prisoners were being evaluated by the psychiatric staff at Bellevue could turn into hours. "You could spend a whole shift at the hospital," he remembers, "and it looked like a station house out there." Now, he says, careful work by the hospital and the local precinct has ironed out many of the problems. "I remember when cops always complained about the hospital; now I'm surprised when I hear a complaint. . . . It's a bond. In any stressful situation, both the officer and the hospital staff are under a lot of stress. A bond of understanding develops." There is also a "bond of understanding" between the precinct and the hospital; Butler serves as a troubleshooter, but there are close relationships up and down the police and hospital hierarchies. There are formal meetings between the precinct captain and the hospital administration every two to three months, and informal communications are constant.

At Denver General Hospital, relations between the hospital and the sheriffs who serve it couldn't be much closer, especially physically. Twenty-three sheriffs provide the police presence in the hospital, where their station house is located. When a prisoner is brought in by a police officer or an "outside" sheriff, he is remanded to the custody of the hospital sheriffs at the hospital door, and he remains in their custody as long as he is a patient. Captain Shields E. Ore, the officer in charge of the sheriffs, reports that the system works very well; because of the small number of sheriffs, they come to know the ED staff well, and conflicts are at a minimum. Sheriffs chosen for duty at the hospital are specially trained in legal issues and sensitivity to patients and staff, and they "are selected for common sense, which is the most important thing," according to associate ED director Gordon. "It's a good beat," Ore says. "Sheriffs ask for duty here. And it means that there's no such thing as 'police intrusion' at the hospital." In addition to straight police work and custodial duties, the sheriffs are also responsible for the security of the ED as a whole.

WHO GIVES THE ORDERS?

Glenn Neilson, chief of security for North Central Bronx Hospital, is a former New York City policeman, and he sees in the broad powers that are accorded to police officers the seeds of trouble for some hospitals. "The waters part when the police arrive," he observes dryly. "It's as if the Saviour has come. There's a feeling of 'silent consent' surrounding a policeman, and it's a bad attitude, especially in hospitals. It can lead to lack of communication."

It can, and does, especially when more than one law enforcement authority is involved, according to Scott at Bernalillo County Medical Center. Both the Albuquerque Police Department and the Bernalillo County Sheriff's Office work with the hospital, she says. The problem is that each group has a separate set of procedures, and the competition between them prevents them from consolidating those procedures. Jurisdictional frictions abound, and the losers in the battle are the patients and the hospital. Each of the two law enforcement groups has a totally different set of procedures for rape victims, for example, and the ED staff members must be prepared to gather evidence in two different ways and to keep two different types of records. The situation is complicated by the fact that because the hospital is a part of the University of New Mexico (UNM), the UNM police also work at the hospital. Actually, Scott reports, the hospital's relations with the UNM police are excellent. There is frequent contact, and most ED staff members and UNM officers are on a first-name basis. But the jurisdictional problems can be confounding. If a crime is committed at the hospital, for example, the Albuquerque police must be called, although the UNM police can hold a suspect for the municipal police.

Scott's main complaint, aside from the confusing array of uniforms and procedures, is that officers who are not from UNM can be, and have been, insensitive to patients at times, although they have shown themselves to be skilled at crisis intervention. The frictions that arise come from a classic conflict: police trying to do their jobs and hospital employees trying to do theirs. Scott describes the unresolved question as being "Is the hospital a place where you enforce the law, or is it a place where you take care of sick people?"

At Auburn Faith Community Hospital, McGlaughlin faced similar problems when the county hospital closed, and his voluntary facility started admitting and treating prisoners and suspects. "By and large," he says, "what I observed was that the sheriffs who worked with the county hospital functioned with the hospital staff as colleagues. They were all part of the system. The sheriffs expected the staff to operate as an extension of the sheriff's department, especially in terms of doing body searches."

At Auburn Faith Community Hospital, staff members would not conduct searches, nor would they follow orders given by sheriffs. It took some time for the sheriffs to adjust to this different environment. "It's been a matter of sitting down and talking with them. They wish we would do more for them, but they understand where we're coming from. There have been ongoing negotiations. If we're not talking with them every three or four months, we should be. The potential for misunderstanding is too great." Things are going smoothly at the moment, McGlaughlin reports, but some frictions remain. "The basic principle," McGlaughlin concludes, "is that we are not going to do their bidding."

RIDING ALONG

Despite such problems, hospital relations with police seem to be improving, largely as a result of hard work by all of those involved. At Lincoln Hospital, Alvarado says, "Our relationship with our local precinct is so good that we don't have problems. In our initial discussions with the police, we emphasized that we are in the patient care business, not the police business. Once that was established, there were few problems." Says Clark of Kings County Hospital, "Our relationship with the police is so excellent that I worry about it sometimes."

Even the good relationships can always use a little support. At Providence Hospital, for example, an already close relationship between Oakland police officers and ED staff members was improved greatly when both sides started talking about the fact that although police officers could watch the ED staff work, the reverse wasn't true. A "ride-along" program was the result: on an individual basis, six nurses, one LVN, and one nursing attendant from the hospital rode along in a police squad car during a shift.

Sergeant Dave Nishihara of the Oakland police reports, "It served two purposes. It gave the nurses a better idea of what we do in the field, and how we have to perform—we have to provide emergency care until the ambulance arrives. Secondly, the nurses provided us with advice on emergency patient care—how to check for bleeding, the color and amount of blood, and so forth." Nishihara is now carrying abdominal pressure pads in his squad car after his "ride-along" nurse partner pointed out their usefulness in emergency situations. Linda Kearney, R.N., day-shift charge nurse for the ED, says, "It gave us more insight into *their* stress, an opportunity to see what they have to deal with."

At Kings County Hospital, ED staff members make a point of treating injured police officers as priority cases; one such officer, waiting to have his broken foot put in a cast, smiles and says, "They're so great here at this hospital!" At Denver General Hospital, employees on coffee break can be found at the sheriff's station, drinking coffee and watching the Denver Broncos on the sheriffs' television set. At Bernalillo County Hospital, Cheryl Scott expresses her admiration for the work of the University of New Mexico police, adding that "without them we'd be up the creek without a paddle."

It seems that the "bond of understanding" that forms between individual police officers and hospital employees is the bottom line, the element that makes these relationships survive the difficult and trying circumstances to which they are often subjected. "It's a 'public safety kinship'," Ira Clark says. "Everything else rests on that." And although he has worked very hard to produce the excellent institutional relationship between his hospital and the local precinct, he says, "I'm proudest of the informal arrangements. They are what feed and strengthen the formal arrangements. If that camaraderie isn't there, then things won't work at 3 a.m. in the emergency department, when all the people who write the formal memos are home in bed."

Chapter 9

Hospital Planning Can Cut Risks of Admitting Prisoner Patients

Barbara Conwell, M.B.A.

The prisoner patient brings to mind the grim prison infirmary seen in old James Cagney movies. But, in fact, it is the modern acute care hospital that often finds itself treating persons under police or prison custody. For this reason, hospital administrators should give some thought to the peculiar hazards and liabilities accompanying the care of prisoner patients. Administrators need to examine some of the potential dangers that the care of prisoner patients may present to other patients, and they need to evolve some guidelines for action to protect the general patient population from harm and the hospital from tort liability.

There are two classes of prisoner patients. Each presents different problems to the hospital. One is the inmate of a prison or jail, who is referred to the hospital because he needs more care than the prison infirmary is able to provide. In this situation, the hospital has the resources of the referring authority to draw on for information regarding the patient's prior history, mental state, and propensity toward violence.

The other type of prisoner patient is the person under police custody, possibly following recent arrest, about whom little is known or disclosed to the hospital. This type of patient often comes into the emergency department in a belligerent mental state, following possible abuse of alcohol or drugs, and probably a short time away from a violent or stressful encounter with the police. He may have been injured in the course of an attempted crime or in the course of his arrest, or he may have been stricken with a serious medical condition during or after his arrest. Delirium tremens and other seizure disorders are frequent medical conditions of prisoner patients who are brought to hospital emergency departments. In situations like this, it is often difficult to obtain reliable information regarding the patient's mental state

Reprinted, with permission, from HOSPITALS, published by the American Hospital Association, copyright November 16, 1978, Vol. 52, No. 22.

and propensity for violence. Such a prisoner has probably been under police observation for only a short time, and the persons transporting him to the hospital may not have witnessed his earlier behavior. The arrestee patient is probably potentially more dangerous than the inmate patient, and he is certainly more difficult to plan for.

Admission of a prisoner patient adds two elements to the usual standard of care required of the hospital in relation to the other patients. The hospital must consider the foreseeability of possible violent or harmful behavior on the part of the prisoner patient, and must take reasonable steps to protect the other patients. In addition, the hospital must take into consideration the reduced capacity of most of the patients. They are unable to provide for their own safety because of their illness, the medication they have taken, or their postoperative condition. This requires that the hospital provide greater safety precautions for regular patients in relation to prisoner patients than would be required in a nonhospital environment.

Most of the case law regarding these extra elements of care relate to the care of mental patients, but there are persuasive analogies to the care of the prisoner. The case of *Schoff v. the State of New York*, 169 N.Y.S. 2d, 245, presented the following fact situation. A 10-year-old boy was admitted to the Rochester State Hospital with a diagnosis of childhood schizophrenia. He was unrestrained by the hospital and was permitted to go freely about the wards and day room. One day he pushed an 84-year-old senile patient with his hands. The octogenarian fell and sustained a fractured femur, among other injuries. The elderly patient's representatives brought suit against the state as the administrator of the state hospital for the injuries sustained. Testimony introduced at the trial supported two key issues—foreseeability and the higher standard of care due to the infirm. The boy was known by hospital staff to be highly excitable, physically active, and impulsive. Although there was no proof that he had ever run into or pushed other patients before, it was foreseeable that his proclivities might lead to such an accident. Thus, it was the hospital's responsibility to control the child appropriately. The hospital staff knew that the elderly patient suffered from arthritis, had difficulty walking and standing, and was somewhat unsteady on his feet. Because he was not able to provide for his own safety, the court ruled that the hospital owed him greater protection from hazardous conditions. The court of appeals upheld the awarding of damages based on the hospital's negligence.

HAZARDOUS SITUATIONS

There are three types of hazardous situations that could arise surrounding the care of the prisoner patient: the prisoner patient could harm other patients directly, either physically or mentally; hospital employees, such as security personnel, could harm a patient as a result of security activities; or a guard, not in the employ of the hospital, could injure another patient.

It is obvious that if bodily harm is done to the victim of a prisoner patient there is a potential tort liability on the part of the hospital, but it is not necessary that bodily harm be inflicted for there to be legal grounds on the part of the victim to seek redress.

A prudent hospital must guard against the likelihood of physical harm and the possibility of shock and terror being inflicted on the nonprisoner patient. These possibilities multiply when prisoner patients of known violent proclivities and their armed or unarmed guards are present in the hospital.

What is the likely course of events if, despite the precautions taken to control the hazards and to protect the general patient population, an incident occurs in which a patient is injured because of the actions of a prisoner patient, his guards, or hospital security personnel. If the victim chooses to bring suit against the hospital, he is likely to petition on the basis of corporate negligence or *respondeat superior.*

Of these, corporate negligence is most likely to be used as a basis for petition. The injured patient would have to prove that the hospital had a duty to provide for his safety, allowing for a possibly weakened capacity on his own part, against reasonably foreseeable hazards under the control of the hospital. He would also have to prove that duty was breached, that harm to himself resulted from that breach, and that the harm was causally related to the breach.

If an injury is caused by a hospital employee, for example, a security guard engaged in a scuffle with a prisoner patient, the victim could bring suit under the doctrine of *respondeat superior,* holding the hospital responsible for the actions of its employee.

When preparing a defense against such actions, the hospital should first examine its statutory immunity status, if any. County and municipal hospitals are the most likely to have standing contracts with prisons to provide care to prisoner patients and may see the largest proportion of such patients. In many cases, these institutions will be covered by immunity statutes. Immunity, however, is coming under fire in some jurisdictions and should not be relied upon absolutely.

The hospital should also examine the issue of comparative negligence when preparing a defense. This issue is especially useful in a situation where the person causing the harm was not employed by the hospital. For example, comparative negligence might be invoked in the event that an injury occurred while the prisoner patient was under the supervision of a prison official or police officer who would presumably have a duty to prevent the prisoner from harming others. Hospitals should be aware of local laws regarding such situations, since comparative negligence laws have not been adopted in all jurisdictions.

Hospitals should also examine the standard of care established in their jurisdiction. As a rule, the hospital would not be held responsible for insuring against remote hazards or against hazards that could not reasonably be foreseen.

RECOMMENDATIONS

The best way to prevent patients from filing suits for damages caused by prisoner patients or their guards is to prevent such injuries from happening. Every hospital that admits prisoner patients or treats arrestee patients in its emergency department should develop a sound policy of risk management to minimize hazards.

The key to risk management of prisoner patients lies in having policies and procedures, preferably in writing, that make the role and responsibility of each employee in the hospital clear. From admission to discharge, procedures should be defined. When a prisoner is admitted, whether as an elective admission or as an emergency case, a responsible individual on the administrative staff (the on-call administrator, for example) should be notified immediately. The administrator should contact the authorities responsible for the detention of the prisoner and obtain clear answers to specific questions. The administrator should find out the exact legal status of the prisoner, whether he is free to leave the hospital, when his medical condition permits, or whether he must be discharged to the authorities, and who may determine his eligibility for leaves of absence.

The administrator should ask about the prisoner's state of mind, whether or not he has shown violent proclivities, and if there are any particular types of people to whom he might be dangerous. If he was an arrestee, the administrator should find out the circumstances of his arrest, and whether or not there was violence, or an indication of drug or alcohol abuse. Finally, the administrator needs to determine whether there will be guards present, if they will be armed, and what arrangements have been made to relieve the guards, or to provide security if no guards are being posted.

The responsible administrator should coordinate the placement of the prisoner patient, taking into consideration the above information. It is highly desirable to have a segregated prison ward, if it is possible, where contact with other patients is minimal. If that is not possible, the prisoner patient should be placed in a private room with a private bath. The patients in nearby rooms should be evaluated so that persons suffering nervous conditions, or who, for other reasons, might be vulnerable as a result of contact with prisoners or guards, can be moved or otherwise kept separate from the prisoner.

If the prisoner is treated in the emergency department, but is not admitted to the hospital, arrangements should be made to have hospital security personnel on hand for the entire time that the prisoner is present. This precaution should be taken even if little is known about the prisoner patient's history prior to his arrival in the hospital.

If the detaining authorities plan to provide guards, accommodations for the guards must be made. These would include provisions for meals and toilet facilities. A hospital policy decision must be made on whether the guards may carry weapons or firearms. If weapons are permitted, appropriate provisions must be made for the safety of the staff and the other patients. It is better for the hospital if the detaining authorities provide their own guards. This provision reduces the hospital's security staffing obligations and provides the shared responsibility necessary for a legal defense of comparative negligence, if any suits should be filed. On the other hand, hospital administrators should consider the presence of armed guards as a dangerous situation and they should weigh the risks and benefits of such a situation in each case.

The administrator assigned to the prisoner patient should be notified by the nursing and medical staff if there is any significant change in the patient's condition or if he needs to be moved to another location. Reminders concerning this procedure should be made in the prisoner patient's chart or on the nursing cardex. The same administrator should also clear any plans for predischarge, leave of absence, and access of visitors to the prisoner patient. It is the administrator's responsibility to provide for the safety of the general patient population and to cooperate with the detaining authorities in their legitimate concerns.

Hospitals can also find themselves in delicate positions regarding the rights of the prisoner himself, including questions of habeas corpus, methods of obtaining evidence, and issues concerning testimony. Therefore, it is doubly desirable that a member of the administrative team take responsibility for all aspects of the care of a prisoner patient, so that inappropriate decisions are not made haphazardly by lower level staff.

LONG-TERM PLANNING

Besides the need for administrative responsibility on the part of the hospital during a prisoner patient's stay, there is also a need for long-term planning and training in the proper methods of handling prisoner patients. If the frequency of admissions warrants it, physical renovations should be considered so that a segregated prison ward or a secure private room is provided. Policy guidelines should be issued and explained to all staff members who might come into contact with a prisoner patient. A coordinated approach to a prisoner's stay, with a single individual identified as the administrator responsible for decisions and planning related to the prisoner, is invaluable.

Finally, the hospital's general liability insurance should be reviewed to ensure that its provisions cover all contingencies related to the care of prisoner patients. If a hospital has a substantial number of prisoner patients, the insurance company would probably be willing to assist hospital administrators in developing a program of risk management planning.

Chapter 10

Hostage Incidents in Health Care Settings

James T. Turner, Ph.D.

The image of care giving and life saving in health care settings is being marred by the reflection of the violent society in which we live. Shootings, assaults, and robberies are becoming facts of daily life in hospital environments. Headlines scream at this:

- Mental patient arrested after shooting spree (Dallas, 1983)
- Nurse guilty of murdering 12 patients (California, 1981)
- Gunman surrenders after hostage drama at hospital (Wyoming, 1982)
- Nurse stays calm while held hostage (Florida, 1983)
- Terrorism strikes the vulnerable (Georgia, 1982)

A phenomenon arising from the criminal and political terrorist activities is now appearing in medical environments—hostage taking. The seizing of hostages has become a popular crime for the powerless throughout the world. Victims range from specific individuals to airplane loads of random victims. United State intelligence sources indicate that $150 million in ransom for hostage takings and kidnapping was paid last year. Unfortunately, the trend continues.

In the 1980s, no health care setting appears safe from hostage incidents. I have been able to identify 22 hostage-taking incidents since late 1981. (Significantly, no central registry for such incidents exists.) The list of targeted medical settings includes a wide variety of environments: general hospitals, outpatient clinics, admissions areas, nursing care units, children's hospitals, and dialysis units. The cities involved are widespread, and include New York, Biloxi, Memphis, Ft. Worth, New Orleans, Laramie, and Los Angeles. Small as well as large cities are targets: Granite City, Ashland, Ft. Lyon.

Hostage taking involves the act of securing total control over a human being for the purpose of ensuring compliance with a pledge made by those interested in, or obligated to, securing the victim's redemption.[1] The value of the hostage's life and physical integrity is interposed as a shield between the hostage taker and those who would rescue the hostage. Hostage taking is not new. However, since 1967, with the advent of urban guerilla movements, hostage taking has gained ascendence in terms of perceived threat and media attention. As hostage taking is a form of political rhetoric for terrorists too weak to cause revolution, so in many cases hostage takings in health care are the acts of those feeling powerless in relation to the health care system. They need to be heard and demand to have their perceived needs met.

In this chapter, I shall examine some of the specific incidents that have affected health care settings. In general, political terrorism has had a minimal impact on health care settings. The only act clearly linked to terrorism is the 1981 slaying of the director of the health care system in Italy. Political terrorists claimed responsibility for this assassination.[2] Most hostage takings in health care settings have occurred as a result of criminals in treatment, psychiatric illness, or emotional disturbance.

THE INCIDENTS

I have detailed elsewhere some of the steps that can be taken to understand and manage health care-based incidents.[3,4,5] Here, I will review several selected incidents to provide an overview and an understanding of the variety of such incidents. It is worth noting that many hospitals are reluctant to provide information on such incidents. One hope is that after examining accounts of these incidents, administrators and victims will step forward with information. In this way, a better understanding of the causes and patterns of these incidents can be developed.

New York, October 1982:[6,7] At around 11 a.m., a convicted robber grabbed a guard's weapon, shot the guard, and took five hospital employees hostage. The siege lasted 46.5 hours with nonstop negotiations. Mr. V., the robber, presented one of the most seasoned negotiation units with one of its longest and most dangerous incidents.

He demanded blankets, pillows, and cigarettes. He wanted to talk with a cousin and the media and demanded to be transferred to a federal correctional institution. When he failed to get the media coverage, or when he was unsatisfied with news accounts, his behavior became extremely threatening. The lives of the hostages many times appeared to hinge on his rapport with the negotiators. This rapport was often the only barrier to violent action.

The 1,200-bed hospital, which also handles 2,000 clinic visits a day, was able to maintain services without interruption.

Newspaper accounts indicate that Mr. V. was able to take the guard's gun after a cast had been removed from his hand, even though the hand was bandaged and in a sling and his other wrist was manacled with a leg iron. Another guard reportedly held the manacle. Mr. V. fired a shot, hitting one guard in the arm. A second shot missed the other guard. Mr. V. raced to the employees' locker room, where he took his hostages.

The five hostages, all male, endured the ordeal for different lengths of time and with varying levels of stress. Six individuals actually were held, but one was released immediately to inform the police that Mr. V. had hostages. This is not an unusual occurrence. Released hostages provide valuable information (often referred to as intelligence) on the situation inside the hostage area, including descriptions and locations of the hostages and the hostage taker.

Three of the five hostages were released during the first day of the incident. Approximately five hours after the hostage taking (4:10 p.m.), a fifty-six-year-old messenger was traded for a variety of comfort items such as blankets and pillow. At 9 p.m., about ten hours into the incident, a second hostage, an office aide, was released after a statement written by Mr. V. was read over a local radio station. A third hostage, an instructional aide, was released at 11:30 p.m. after Mr. V. was satisfied with the 11 o'clock news coverage. In exchange for the fourth hostage, a hospital barber who was not released until 4:30 p.m. the next day, Mr. V. was allowed to tape radio and television interviews explaining his position.

Negotiations for the fifth hostage collapsed after Mr. V. realized his television interview had been edited. Thirty-six hours into the incident, he was enraged, tired, and demanding live air time on all the local television stations. His moods changed rapidly and ranged from exhilaration to rage. He threatened the hostages with Russian roulette, and negotiators became concerned about his suicide potential.

The rapport between the police negotiators and Mr. V. was extremely important in ending the siege. Significant problems developed over his depiction by the media, and technical problems delayed the promised television broadcast. Finally, a deputy corrections commissioner was able to relay Mr. V.'s latest statement on live television. At about 8:30 a.m., the last hostage, an office aide, appeared to the applause of the crowd. In the end, Mr. V. surrendered to the authorities. The 46.5-hour siege was over and everyone was safe.

Fort Worth, Texas, September 1982:[8,9,10] Mr. B., a twenty-four-year-old nonpatient, seized four hostages on a locked psychiatric ward at approximately 8 p.m. Mr. B.'s actions were related to his delusions of a break-up with a "girlfriend." He thought somehow his hostage taking would reunite them. This siege lasted for 17 hours. While 20 patients were evacuated, a number of patients were cut off from the police. The hostage taker, in the steel-walled nursing station, was between the police and the patient group.

Mr. B received hamburgers, and demanded to see various members of his family and his girlfriend, who had actually had been merely an acquaintance seven years before.

The first hostage was released early in the incident. This male nursing assistant talked Mr. B. into letting him leave to keep hospital security officials from storming the area. At 11:30 p.m., two hostages, a male nursing assistant in his twenties and a Latin-American female in her thirties, were released. At that point, two hostages remained, a licensed vocational nurse (L.V.N.) in her thirties and a registered nurse (R.N.) in her twenties.

At around 1 a.m., the L.V.N. was exchanged for food. This left the R.N. alone in the steel-walled nursing station. According to interviews with the R.N. in the *Star-Telegraph*, Mr. B. put the gun to her head at times, to which she would respond, "I wish you wouldn't point it at me." The R.N. spent much of her time trying to keep Mr. B. from becoming too upset. At 1 p.m. the next day, she convinced Mr. B. to allow her to leave the room for a cup of ice. The R.N.'s clear impression was that Mr. B. wanted to die. She clearly remembered the beginning as the worst part of the 17-hour ordeal. "We didn't know how he'd act. We were scared he'd start shooting at any little thing we did." She reported talking and joking with him. She was also able to get some sleep. The police finally assaulted Mr. B. when the R.N. went to check the ice machine for the second time. The firing began. Mr. B. surrendered.

The staff found the nursing station in a mess—14 bullet holes, papers, and coffee cups. A portable blood pressure machine had been hit. The unit had to be closed, and arrangements had to be made to send involuntary patients elsewhere. Reviews of procedure were necessary. Would the staff come back? How much time off and overtime pay would the hostages receive?

New Orleans, Louisiana, November 1981:[11,12] A patient armed with a .38-caliber rifle held the hospital director hostage for more than four hours. He apparently was upset over a cut in his disability payments. He took the director hostage to air his anger and because the director was a symbol of government indifference. Mr. X. walked into the director's office suite, suggested that the secretaries take their lunch breaks, and then entered the director's office. All 20 staff members in the area were evacuated immediately. About two hours later, the main lobby was also evacuated. A lapse in time occurred before the local police were called. This resulted from a jurisdictional issue; the federal facility notified the Federal Bureau of Investigation first and then decided to call in local resources, a Special Weapons and Tactics (SWAT) team and a negotiation team.

The negotiators were able to use the man's relationship with his family to break the siege mentality. They convinced him that his family would suffer if he died. He surrendered with no shots fired and no injuries. The hostage taker was sentenced to three years in jail.

New Orleans, Louisiana, January 31, 1982:[13,14] A thirty-one-year-old male stormed the outpatient treatment area with a .22-gauge, double-barreled shotgun at 9:30 a.m., taking two patients, two physicians, and two assistants hostage. He soon released all but one, a forty-year-old male nurse. The incident lasted for approximately three hours, during which the patient reported being upset after reading about a veteran who committed suicide earlier that week because no one would give him any help. Mr. C. repeatedly told police he wanted to die. He wanted them to kill him when they attempted to rescue the hostage. The hostage was allowed to talk to the police on the telephone and provided police with significant information about room size, physical conditions, and weapons. The negotiators sought to convince Mr. C. that someone did care and that his life was worth saving. In addition to his demand to die, Mr. C. demanded that his brother be brought to the hospital. The final hostage was released at approximately 12:10 p.m. A tense period followed, as negotiators feared he would commit suicide. At 12:25 p.m., he surrendered. Mr. C. was convicted and sentenced to ten years in jail.

Lake Butler, Florida, May 1983:[15] A female R.N. was held hostage by a thirty-year-old state prison inmate who broke away from a corrections officer. The inmate grabbed her around the neck and threatened to kill her with a sharpened toilet plunger. He demanded drugs and told the R.N. he wanted to be killed by members of the department of corrections. The incident lasted 45 minutes.

The R.N. used medication to keep her captor from killing himself while the officers tried to negotiate with him. She administered enough Valium and Demerol to make him drowsy. When he began displaying the effects of the drugs, four officers rushed and subdued him after a brief struggle. The R.N. planned to return to work after two days off.

Laramie, Wyoming, September 1982:[16,17] A twenty-nine-year-old man held 10 to 15 people hostage in a hospital center for two hours. The man entered the hospital at about 10:45 a.m. through the emergency room carrying a Ruger .22-caliber semi-automatic carbine and 500 rounds of ammunition; he proceeded to the mental health center on the second floor.

At first, the employees thought it was a joke. Mr. Y. fired one shot into the ceiling. Most of the persons left the area. A family consultant remained with the hostage taker, but left after talking with Mr. Y. for 20 minutes. The reasons for the incident are somewhat confused. After the police allowed Mr. Y. to talk with his ex-wife, he surrendered. Some disruption of outpatient services occurred; x-ray and laboratory work was slowed as these work areas were in the police-secured area. Hospital security sealed the area, relocated some staff members and patients, and turned the incident over to the local SWAT team.

Woodland, California, September 1983:[18] Mr. S., thirty-one, held 15 hospital employees for 90 minutes. He took over the hospital cafeteria with a double-barreled shotgun and fired one shot into the ceiling. The incident lasted for approximately three hours. Mr. S. demanded to be given information related to the health of his son. In August, Mr. S. had been admitted to the hospital's psychiatric ward for evaluation. The hostages escaped after being held for two and one-half hours while Mr. S. talked to a police negotiator. He surrendered 30 minutes later.

Los Angeles, California, August 1983:[19,20] A gunman who claimed to be on an anti-abortionist mission from God held hostage two women employees of a center offering reproductive medical services. The incident lasted for 14 hours and may have been motivated by revenge against the clinic's head physician. Supposedly, the physician had seen the man's wife and had been threatened by the hostage taker.

During the incident, the gunman made several demands, including transportation. He allowed one of the hostages, a receptionist, to talk with her husband. The other hostage was a female medical assistant. He threatened to kill the hostages as he followed the incident on radio and television. At one point, he called a local television station and talked with a reporter. Fourteen hours after the incident began, he tried to run with the hostages to a car using a smoke screen from a fire extinguisher. The police shot him to death. One of the hostages was wounded in the leg.

Memphis, Tennessee, February 1982:[21] A lone gunman with a .357-Magnum handgun took four people hostage. This drama, which was to last 34 hours, involved a male psychiatrist, a male pediatric cancer physician, a female psychological examiner, and a female registered nurse. Mr. G. walked into St. Jude's before 10:30 a.m., taking the psychological examiner hostage first. The examiner then called the other three staff members to her offices, fearing that if she did not, Mr. G. would go to the primary treatment area that was filled with children. Mr. G. was the father of a child who had died at the hospital. His goals were to make a scandal for the hospital and to be taken to the room on the sixth floor where his son had died. He also wanted live television coverage. Police negotiators feared he would kill the hostages and then himself on television. Police negotiators required that he give up his gun before being allowed to go to the sixth floor as it was "sacred" ground, but he refused. For 24 hours, this demand was repeated. At 4:15 p.m., the elderly psychiatrist was allowed to go for food. Police quickly took him and refused to allow him to return, even though he strongly protested.

Finally, Mr. G. demanded a radio broadcast. He revealed that for more than three years he had been trying to get someone—public health officials, physicians, the Drug Enforcement Agency, and the Federal Drug Administration—to listen to his theory of leukemia. No one would listen until now. His radio broadcast related his theory: he had had hepatitis, and his wife had been given the drug DES during pregnancy. These two factors, according to Mr. G., were responsible for the child's cancer.

Mr. G. repeatedly threatened the hostages, putting the .357 in their backs and cocking the hammer. He also handcuffed two of them together, placed the .357 at the physician's back, and told them that if he fired, the bullet would go through both of them.

The hospital faced a number of problems: continuing services that no other hospital could provide, maintaining crowd control, and providing information to the hostages' families. A number of the preparedness issues that I have addressed in the manual *Management and Understanding of Hostage Incidents in Healthcare* (P. O. Box 17781, Memphis, Tennessee 31817-0781) were important factors in the management of the incident.[3]

At one point, the hostage taker placed the gun on a table and began to leave with the hostages. However, he stated he felt a hand pulling him back into the room. At this point, he appears to have experienced a full psychotic break. He began saying sentences backwards and experiencing olfactory hallucinations. Approximately 34 hours into the incident, a Tactical Apprehension Containment Team (TACT) began moving into place for an assault. The physician lunged at Mr. G. and began struggling for the weapon. Police burst through the door. As Mr. G. hissed, "I'll kill you, you son of a bitch," an officer pulled the trigger on the M-16, killing Mr. G. No hostages were physically injured.

The incidents described above represent only a sampling of more than 20 incidents since 1981 of which I have been aware. These examples provide a glimpse into a type of action that strikes all types of health care facilities.

HOSTAGE TAKERS IN HEALTH CARE

Thomas Strentz in his chapter reviews personality types and categories of mental disorders. In this section, I want to examine hostage takers thematically, rather than by personality types or on a mental-disorders basis. A recurring theme throughout the hostage takings in health care settings is a lack of power. Hostage taking is the crime of the weak and powerless. One individual can gain the attention of local media, the government, and possibly the nation. The individual can go from being unheard and shunned to having a powerful audience hanging on every word. The rise of health care as a bureaucratic institution and the decline of the life-to-death physician and nurse models lead more people to feel ignored and uncared for in terms of emotional and coping needs. Two categories of hostage takers first identified by H. H. A. Cooper[22] are the aggrieved person and the estranged person.

Aggrieved individuals feel that they have legitimate grievances that no one in a position of responsibility will address. Often such individuals have made numerous attempts to get a response from the system. In most cases, the organization not only refuses to correct the perceived wrong, but also implies that the individual has no basis for a complaint. After exhausting multiple system options—the media, hospitals, governmental agencies—the individual feels driven to the dramatic. In this way, feelings of helplessness are pushed away, and, in fact, people do listen. As pointed out by Thomas Strentz, many times negotiators discover that the primary goal of the hostage taker is to be heard by someone of importance.

Health care institutions in many cases have become impersonal bureaucracies that present an indifferent organizational front. The opportunities to fail to listen increase and the feeling of powerlessness among patients, families, and the community increases.

The second thematic group likely to place health care settings in the crossfire is the estranged individual. These persons are separated from, or on the verge of losing, significant figures in their lives. With those relationships impaired, for whatever reason, the hostage takers seek to coerce the maintainance of those relationships through forceful action. Police negotiators are familiar with the individuals (usually males) who barricade themselves with their families and hold the police at bay while threatening suicide and/or death to the family members unless the family members relent from certain courses of action.

Health care settings become battlegrounds where such incidents are played. Children are placed in hospitals for court-mandated treatment. An estranged parent is forbidden to see a child, even when the child is hospitalized. A father holds staff members hostage to force administrators to provide information about his child's health. A man seeks through force to speak with his ex-wife, who is receiving medical care. A man tries to storm a hospital with weapons and bombs to free his wife from court-ordered psychiatric care. Examples abound where people are separated from each other in the medical setting. Hostage taking becomes a means to force the reestablishment of those relationships.

STAFF TRAINING

Staffs usually perform while they train. As discussed in John Moran's chapter, reduction of injury and better management of aggressive behavior occurs when the staff takes the responsibility for managing such behaviors. This responsibility demands training in preventing and managing such behavior. In hostage incidents, such training can literally spell the difference between life or death, between a minor incident and a lengthy hostage taking. Hostage survival training, as discussed by Thomas Strentz, is one element in such training. Additional areas for training include procedures for the first person on the scene and basic negotiation skills. Many hospital administrators and service delivery professionals have the mistaken idea that someone else will take care of these incidents. My review of such incidents indicates that response time of the appropriate outside authorities ranged from ten minutes to two hours. The events of the first five to ten minutes are not only some of the most dangerous, but they also set the stage for what is to come, based on the professional staff's actions. Serious errors that may cost the lives of staff members, patients, visitors or the hostage taker can be made if health care staffs are not trained to respond during those initial minutes.

ADMINISTRATIVE ISSUES

Accreditation standards direct the development of crisis plans for many kinds of disasters. Earthquakes, fires, and hostage-taking incidents occur frequently enough that they merit consideration in preparing crisis plans. Disaster plans require particular types of information. This section briefly summarizes a few of those issues discussed elsewhere in greater detail.[3]

ADMINISTRATIVE ORGANIZATION

An administrative plan needs to include provisions for a clear line of command and control. No question should arise in the mind of the first employee on the scene as to whom notice is to be given. A specific person (or persons) should be authorized to begin the notification process within the hospital. Policy should clearly define whether or not the police are to be called at the initial contact. If not, what office is responsible for making the contact with the designated person within the police department?

The initial person on the scene needs to understand that orders given under duress are not to be followed except to save lives, and that no deals can be made by employees.

Additionally, the plan should specify individuals authorized to set aside areas for police command posts, a negotiator area, and a resource area. An information officer also should be designated by the plan.

In most cases, the authority designated by the administrative plan must decide whether or not to use internal resources. This decision will be influenced by a number of factors, including jurisdictional issues and the level of training of organization police or security as opposed to that of the local community police authority.

The primary goal at this point in the plan is to contain and stabilize the situation and to establish a command and control structure. The details of such planning are discussed elsewhere.[3]

STAFF IMPACT

Health care settings need to plan for coping with the impact of hostage incidents. The reactions of both the victims and other staff members can lead to quality of care issues.

A decision must be made as to how mundane matters such as overtime, time off after the incident, and fitness for return to work will be determined. Hostages may go through many emotional experiences that influence both work and family life. Hostages may feel as if they failed professionally, either by not preventing the incident or by failing to save the hostage taker. Some may be confused and embarrassed by feelings arising from the Stockholm Syndrome—a feeling of empathy for the hostage taker that is incongruent with the victim's situation. Victims may sense that they've been abandoned by those in power and feel confused over their attachment to an individual (the hostage-taker) who has placed their lives in danger.[23]

A significant number of the victims will experience post-traumatic stress syndromes—anxiety, jumpiness when approached, sleep disorders, and vague psychosomatic symptoms. Health care settings need to provide confidential sources of treatment and to inform victims of any requirements, such as physical examinations for insurance purposes or depositions for the record.

Bursten et al.[24] examined the generalized impact of a hostage taking on uninvolved staff members. It is clear that the increase in post-traumatic stress symptoms is not limited to the victims. Organized discussion groups that focus on information and sharing are quite useful.

SUMMARY

No facility appears safe from hostage-taking incidents. Increased security and staff training can make these acts more difficult to commit. However, as a result of the inherent openness of the health care setting, it appears to be impossible to completely prevent such incidents. Plans for managing hostage-taking incidents are essential and can also be applied to a number of different human crisis situations.

NOTES

1. R. W. Kobetz and H. H. Cooper, *Target Terrorism* (Gaithersburg, Md: International Association of Chiefs of Police, 1978).

2. Y. Alexander and R. S. Cline, eds., "Worldwide Chronology of Terrorism—1981," *Terrorism* 6 (1982): 246-247.

3. J. T. Turner, ed., *Management and Understanding of Hostage Incidents in Healthcare* (Memphis: LifeStyle Management Associates, Inc., 1984).

4. J. T. Turner, "The Role of the ED Nurse in Health-Care Based Hostage Incidents," *The Journal of Emergency Nursing*, July/August 1984, in press.

5. Interview of J. T. Turner in writing a hostage-taking response plan, *Hospital Security and Safety Management* 4 (1983): 5-10.

6. J. P. Fried, "Convict Holding Two as Hostages Inside a Hospital," *New York Times*, October 15, 1982.

7. D. W. Dunlap, "Gunman Frees Last of Five Hostages and Surrenders," *New York Times*, October 17, 1982.

8. G. Bailon, "Former Patient Demands Talks with Four People," *Star-Telegram*, September 17, 1982.

9. E. Harrison, "JPS Was Prepared for Worst in Ordeal," *Star-Telegram*, September 18, 1982.

10. D. Ferman, "Nurse Recalls JPS Ordeal," *Short Horn*, September 22, 1982.

11. B. Dansker, "Veteran Holds Hospital Chief Hostage Four Hours," *Times-Picayune*, November 14, 1981.

12. E. Anderson, "Man Who Held VA Chief Hostage Receives Three-year Sentence," *Times-Picayune*, May 20, 1982.

13. B. Dansker, "Man Surrenders at VA Hospital," *Times-Picayune*, February 1, 1982.

14. B. Dansker, "Tough Task for Negotiator: Gain Trust of Hostage-taker," *Times-Picayune*, February 7, 1982.

15. A. DeLotto, "Nurse Stays Calm While Held Hostage," *Florida Nursing News*, May 14, 1983.

16. R. Roten, "Gunman Surrenders After Hostage Drama at Hospital," *The Boomerang*, September 22, 1982.

17. P. Wolfinbarger, "Hospital Plan Works Well," *The Boomerang*, September 22, 1982.

18. R. C. Paddock, "Deputy Kills Gunman as Twenty Hostages Hide in Film Lab; Two Other Suspects Captured," *Los Angeles Times*, September 23, 1983.

19. D. Hastings and P. Morrison, "Gunman Holds Two Health Clinic Workers Hostage," *Los Angeles Times*, August 3, 1983.

20. D. Hastings and P. Morrison, "Man Slain by Police Linked to Murder," *Los Angeles Times*, August 4, 1983.

21. W. Crews and D. Dawson, "Thirty-four Hours," *Memphis* 7 (1982): 92-103.

22. H. H. A. Cooper, *The Hostage Takers* (Boulder: Palidin Press, 1982).

23. T. Strentz, "The Stockholm Syndrome: Law Enforcement Policy and Ego Defenses of the Hostage," *FBI Law Enforcement Bulletin* 48 (1979): 2-12.

24. B. Bursten et al., "Reducing Stress in a Traumatized Hospital," in *Management and Understanding of Hostage Incidents in Healthcare*, ed. J. Turner (Memphis: LifeStyle Management Associates, Inc., 1984).

Chapter 11

Hostage Survival Guidelines

Thomas Strentz, M.S.W.

THE BANK ROBBERY

At 10:15 a.m. on Thursday, August, 23, 1973, the quiet routine of the Sveriges Kredit Bank in Stockholm, Sweden, was destroyed by the clatter of a Swedish K 9mm submachine gun. As clouds of plaster and glass settled around the 60 stunned occupants, a heavily armed, lone gunman called out in English, "The party has just begun."[1]

The "party" was to continue for 131 hours, permanently affecting the lives of four young hostages and giving birth to a new dimension of study that would be used to prepare potential victims of hostage situations.

INTRODUCTION

An increasing incidence, or at least an increase in the reporting, of both targeted and random hostage situations has underscored the psychological and physical needs of victims and potential victims of hostage situations. Studies conducted thus far have answered some questions, but have raised others.[2,3,4] For instance, how should victims behave to protect their lives? What psychological strategies and training might be employed before an incident to help potential victims cope with a psychologically stressful and life-threatening situation?

Evidence of the value of preparation for potential victims is growing. American law enforcement agencies and banks have learned that tellers who have been trained to cope with the trauma of a robbery or a hostage situation survive such episodes as stronger people. Untrained employees tend to become hysterical and are frequently traumatized by the experience.[5,6]

It is my intent to identify some of the problems faced by hostages, and to suggest courses of action for potential hostages that will enable them to weather the siege. Survival with dignity may enable the former hostage to recover more quickly and return to a normal routine. This chapter will also suggest some precautions that potential victims can take to avoid being taken hostage.

TYPES OF HOSTAGE TAKERS

One way to prepare for the ordeal of being a hostage is to know something about those who take hostages. The three most common types of hostage takers are the criminal subject, the mentally ill subject, and the politically motivated subject.

The Criminal Subject

Antisocial Personality

This individual is usually the armed robber trapped at the crime scene (bank, pharmacy, quick grocery) because of rapid police response. When he learns that the police have him cornered, he takes hostages to secure his escape. The criminal bargains with police in an attempt to keep the money or goods from the robbery, to gain additional funds, and to find a way out of this dilemma and reach freedom. This type of subject can be identified by the logical nature of his demands, for example, money, food, and freedom. The hostages are generally unknown to him. Research has shown that such an individual is an experienced felon and has an above-average education for a criminal.[7]

Inadequate Personality

This individual is the armed robber who, because of poor planning, has seriously miscalculated his ability to rob an establishment. Errors are almost childlike; demands, such as a million dollars in gold, border on the impossible. Unlike the antisocial personality, the inadequate person has a limited history of criminal behavior and his demands are almost apologetic. He may state his demands with considerable conviction and then provide the negotiator with several options. This person may also be a confederate of the leader, a follower, a "goofer"—unpredictable if left to his own devices.

The Mentally Ill Subject

Paranoid Schizophrenic

This is the most common type of mentally ill subject. Demands are frequently bizarre; a bank robber in California demanded that a truckload of birdseed be delivered to every bank in Los Angeles, that everyone in Los Angeles walk to the ocean for a cleansing, and that all vehicles cease movement for two days. He also demanded that the authorities turn off the moon.

Depressed

Another mentally ill subject is the deeply depressed individual who may be suicidal. These individuals can be identified by their quiet tones, slow speech patterns, and negative outlooks. They may kill or give the impression that they have injured a hostage to force the police to shoot them. Demands are generally mixed with statements of depression and references to death. The hostages are frequently known to them. By taking hostages, they are crying out for help; they want to be punished, but they are often willing to be talked out of their plans.

The Politically Motivated Subject

These individuals are rare in the United States, but more common in Europe and South America. They usually select the time, place, and hostages very carefully. They provide the authorities with the greatest challenges and are the most serious threat to the welfare of hostages, since they, more than any others, have executed hostages.

In the United States, there seems to be a dearth of politically motivated individuals who take hostages in an attempt to advance their causes. It may be that most Americans believe that a political hostage situation, such as the taking of Israeli athletes by Black September at Munich in September 1972, is counterproductive. The radical fringe of American politics through our history has had its ideas incorporated by the major political parties. Our dynamic democracy has been responsive to change, and thus has acted to prevent terrorism before it could begin. Or, it may be that since our open society has multiple avenues for the expression of political convictions, those who resort to the taking of hostages to further political aims are labeled as mentally ill, rather than taken seriously as political actors.[9] However, in some countries, as a Rand Corporation study clearly indicates,[2] the majority of hostage situations are perpetrated by those who are politically motivated. This has been verified by a review of the German and Dutch hostage negotiator training manuals that focus on the problem of politically motivated hostage takers. These manuals mention other types of hostage situations only as opportunities for the police to sharpen their negotiating and assault skills.

STAGES OF INTERVENTION

This chapter will focus on primary intervention and will deal with the factors to consider when one is abducted or taken hostage, the stages of hostage situations, and some recovery techniques.

Stephen Auerbach points out that programs designed to assist individuals involved in crises are quite different from standard psychotherapeutic models of intervention.[8] The field of crisis intervention therapy generally deals with basically healthy individuals whose current emotional dysphoria seems to be a function of their response to a specific, reality-oriented stressor—the crisis—with which they are so overburdened that they are temporarily unable to cope.[9]

Auerbach further identifies four types of crisis intervention therapy or programs.

Primary Intervention

This program is designed to acquaint potential victims with knowledge of the crisis they may face to enable them to cope more effectively should they be victimized. Examples of primary intervention include classes on rape prevention for females, management of violent behavior training for health care staffs, prisoner of war training for military pilots, robbery seminars for bank employees, disaster drills for civil defense volunteers, and the various exercises used by the military to prepare for combat experience.

Preparation Intervention

Immediate pre-impact intervention is a program that deals with individuals known to be on the verge of confrontation with a stressful life event. Again, information on what to expect is delivered. For instance, expectant mothers, patients facing surgery, or individuals about to begin dangerous assignments all know that they will be confronted with a stressful event. However, there is a period of time between learning of the occurrence and the actual impact.

Recovery Treatment

Short-term impact intervention is designed to assist recent crisis victims to regain psychological equilibrium. Programs of this type commonly deal with victims of rape and natural disaster, former prisoners of war, certain types of surgery patients, and, most recently, victims of hostage situations.

Long-term Treatment

Long-term post-impact treatment intervention is common in the United States and deals with individuals who have not and cannot recover by themselves from the emotional trauma of a crisis. Any of the above-delineated crisis victims who have not returned to a normal level of social functioning after a few months may be candidates for this type of crisis treatment.[8]

PRIMARY INTERVENTION TECHNIQUES

Prevention

Brooks McClure, a Department of State analyst who has debriefed countless hostages, says that it is wise for vulnerable people to be alert to signs that they are marked for seizure. They might sense that they are being watched; they may catch glimpses of the same people in various parts of town; they may become aware that their cars are being followed.[10]

Brian Jenkins of the Rand Corporation modifies McClure's advice, but agrees with the idea that an ounce of prevention is worth a pound of cure. While fear of being abducted need not become an obsession of the individual, elementary security precautions can be enacted easily. Only a few terrorists have mobilized large numbers of individuals and demonstrated daring in kidnapping a specific targeted individual. Most abductions are carried out by small groups who have selected their targets because of their inattention to safety and security measures.[2]

Kidnappers and hostage takers, like other criminals, are seeking the greatest return for the least amount of effort or risk on their part. Changing routines, altering schedules, taking vacations, traveling with others, or purchasing large dogs are a few of the measures taken by individuals who are being targeted to successfully deter their abductors. The effectiveness of such measures has been measured by interviewing terrorists to determine why certain individuals were selected for abduction over more politically attractive targets.[2]

Sophisticated terrorists do not take unnecessary risks; their dedication is limited. They seek soft targets to maximize success over time and to increase the subsequent propaganda value gained by their acts.

Preparation

The personal preparation for abduction may take many forms. One common avenue is to purchase kidnap insurance. This is a controversial issue. Some authorities contend that if it becomes known that an individual is so insured, the insurance could be an inducement to kidnapping.[11] However, this has been documented only once. The Montoneros, an Argentine terrorist group, learned of a kidnap insurance policy through a company secretary, kidnapped the two brothers who were insured, and demanded a payment equal to the amount of the insurance.[12]

Most companies that issue such policies require that their customers take certain precautions. These acts of precaution also serve as acts of prevention or target hardening. In some cases, they require their clients' chauffeurs to be trained in evasive driving techniques. Clients may be required to vary their commuting routes and desystemize their work schedules. Lower rates may be available to clients who purchase various types of armored vehicles and engage private security forces. Many companies develop and discuss their kidnapping policies with those employees who are potential victims. This practice seems to be particularly effective, because people are more inclined to adhere to a policy they helped to develop.[13]

Another practice is for each victim's company to guarantee as much assistance as possible to the victim's family. The knowledge that their families are well cared for is of great comfort to those held hostage.[14]

Dr. Frank Ochberg, noted psychiatrist and former director of the Michigan Department of Mental Health, says individuals should discuss the potential for abduction and its implications with significant others. They should consider, as concretely as possible, what might happen and the realistic ways of responding to the danger.[9] He says that emotional preparation can be accomplished with some ease and is an effective way to minimize later stress. It may be helpful for members of a family to acknowledge and discuss the feelings of anxiety and depression with which they may have to cope. Those who would be called upon for psychological and social support could be identified in advance. Family members and acquaintances who might not be able to help could also be identified to spare them unnecessary and debilitating guilt.[11]

Health is another crucial factor to consider when coping with stress. Although common sense dictates limitations on physical heroics, physical conditioning is of crucial importance for effective resistance.

More tangible preparations should also be made. Unknown to the abductors, wills should be updated and should convey a great deal of information to the victim's family. A primary advantage of these and other techniques of self-control lies in the psychological benefit that they may offer in an emotional and stressful situation.

Resistance

No one can tell individuals whether they should resist an abductor. This decision must be made by individuals on the basis of their own calculations of the immediate situation, their physical abilities, and the number of subjects they are facing. It is risky to resist. Victims should understand that during the opening moments or the alarm phase of a hostage situation, victims are expendable. Terrorists can create equally effective propaganda from a killing as they can from an abduction. Even though the primary motivation of the criminals may be to abduct, their greatest concern will be their own safety and freedom.

Abduction

Over the years, many studies have been conducted to identify patterns and trends in abductions. According to McClure,[10] there are similarities in the psychological reactions of most individuals to being abducted or taken hostage. It does not matter who the victims are or where they are taken. Hostages will almost always react in a predictable fashion. It helps victims if they understand in advance what their reactions may be.

Being kidnapped is one of the most frightening experiences of a lifetime. Regardless of the length of the period of captivity, victims are under more stress than individuals who are in prison. Kidnap victims may be sentenced to death or they may be released, whereas individuals in prison already know their sentences. The outcome is beyond the kidnap victims' control. And, the time they must wait and wonder before learning of their fate is indefinite and also beyond personal control. The hostage is often alone, yet, according to McClure, the average person's capacity to endure shock, mental stress, and physical abuse is far greater than most would ever expect. With some psychological preparation and an awareness of the innate ability to survive, potential hostages can be fortified and will survive.[10]

THE FOUR STAGES OF A HOSTAGE SITUATION

Through interviews with hostages and a case-by-case evaluation of hostage situations, it appears that hostage situations tend to be divided into four stages. Each phase will be discussed from the vantage point of the subject, the hostage, and law enforcement. Recommendations for hostage survival are also included. Although no specific time frame can be placed upon each stage, certain acts committed by the subjects and the hostages lend themselves to different responses, depending upon the phase of the situation.

The Subject

Alarm

The first and probably most traumatic period is the alarm stage. In many ways, particularly in the case of an armed robbery gone sour, the abductor and the police go through similar experiences.

In desperation, the trapped armed robber compounds his dilemma by adding kidnapping and assault charges. These considerations are initially minimal. Emotions are running high; the hostage taker wants to buy time and succeeds. Research has shown that the leader of the abductors usually has a prior felony arrest.[7] Therefore, though desperate, the hostage taker is not ignorant or inexperienced in the ways of the criminal justice system and realizes the consequences of this action.

The trapped subject is outgunned and outnumbered, and the situation becomes less tenable with each fleeting moment. The subject is now linked with other individuals, usually strangers, who are equally frightened and near panic.

During the alarm stage, the subjects are usually quite aggressive. Subjects become intoxicated on their own hormones and may be shooting at people they believe are police.[15] The subjects are actively engaged in consolidating their rather precarious positions. It is during this stage that the lives of the hostages are in the greatest danger from the subjects. They may be caught in cross fire and accidentally killed.

Even the mentally ill or the political terrorist subject who has planned to take hostages is inclined to be aggressive at this early stage. The subject must force his will upon the hostages quickly to control them and achieve his real purpose. Hostage takers usually want to survive and benefit from their acts. To accomplish this, they must, or think they must, initially terrorize the hostages into total submission. In this endeavor they may be inclined to overreact, to abuse, to threaten, and to harass the hostages. Their reason is diminished due to their high emotional levels.[15]

Crisis

The crisis phase marks the beginning of reason for the hostage taker, yet in many ways it is similar to the alarm phase. The subject is still dangerous and unpredictable.

During the crisis stage, some subjects begin to feel a sense of frustration. If this is an impromptu hostage taking, for example, the outgrowth of a blunder, things will not go as well as the hostage takers would like. Generally, their initial demands reflect this frustration. Hostage takers' early dialogue may be marked by emotional outbursts and excessive demands.

The level of frustration is best indicated by the amount of money demanded. A robber may have expected a few thousand dollars for his efforts at larceny. Once the police have trapped him in the bank, he may believe that he can punish them for this by making them pay a large amount of money. Initial demands for hundreds of thousands of dollars are not unusual. Hostage takers may begin to move the hostages around in an attempt to better secure their positions since they cannot trust anyone and they think a police assault imminent.

The politically motivated hostage taker spends this stage with the hostages. He keeps them busy covering windows with paper or moving furniture and other items around to secure a position. One terrorist group used this time to collect belongings from its hostages. This group took wallets, but returned the money, stating that they were not thieves. Collecting passports, wristwatches, pens, pencils, and other personal belongings from their hostages demonstrates the terrorists' power over their victims. The retaining of personal belongings can also serve as a method of control. Items may later be returned to reward good behavior. So effective was this procedure in the above-mentioned situation that the terrorist group obtained critiques from their hostages as they deplaned.

Mentally ill subjects are also occupied with their concerns for personal safety. However, they do not usually collect personal belongings to control their hostages. Their demands for money do not generally escalate. They begin with outrageous demands, such as a million dollars in gold, or, like Corey Moore in Warrensville Heights, Ohio, that all white people vacate the earth in 24 hours.

Accommodation

This is the longest and most tranquil phase. The reaction of hostage takers during this phase reflects an interest in making the best of a difficult situation. They may bargain with the authorities, or, like the mentally ill hostage taker, they may engage in ventilation.

Mentally ill subjects talk at length with high emotion about problems, ventilate during negotiations, and gradually wind down to an eventual surrender. This type of hostage taker has probably been in a therapy group, has some verbal skills, and is primarily motivated by a need to talk to someone who will listen. Dr. Harvey Schlossberg speaks about this phenomenon when reflecting upon the hundreds of cases he has negotiated. He speaks of the people who want to talk to someone in authority, command attention and who, in fact, fulfill this wish when they hold hostages. Some may miss the attention given them once they are out of the hospital. One of the most experienced FBI negotiators, Bernard Thompson, has had many encounters with hostage takers who, after the initial crisis has passed, just want to talk.

Therefore, throughout the siege, as this type of hostage taker is airing problems and gaining some satisfaction by talking, it becomes apparent that the goal is not escape. The goal is to talk to anyone who will listen.

The criminally motivated subject is not ventilating as much as bargaining. These individuals are trying to strike a deal with the police to achieve their goal of freedom, which results in certain counter tactics by law enforcement officers. These tactics may include, but are not limited to, bargaining with the criminal in a give-and-take atmosphere for several hours, giving the impression that in exchange for the release of hostages, the subject will be allowed freedom. The subject may be given a vehicle as a ploy either to convince him that he will go free or to maneuver him into a position in which the police will be able to control the use of deadly force to terminate the situation without allowing mobility and chancing possible injury to others.

Whereas the mentally ill subject by this stage has completed his ventilation and is in the process of working out the mechanics of surrender, the criminal subject is still bargaining for freedom.

Terrorists, such as the Popular Front for the Liberation of Palestine (PFLP) and the Japanese Red Army (JRA), have taken the time to identify and segregate their hostages during this phase. The PFLP isolated its Israeli hostages in a separate part of the terminal in Entebbe in July 1976, in order to give them "special treatment." It is now believed that even if the government of Israel had complied with the demands of the PFLP and released jailed terrorists, the PFLP had planned to kill the Jewish hostages.

The subjects may gradually make their demands more reasonable because they are beginning to feel the stress of captivity. They may be willing to settle for a face-saving solution, rather than hold out for the initial, and perhaps emotional, demands.

Resolution

This final phase is one of stark contrasts. The mood within and without the siege site depends upon whether the siege is broken by an assault or by surrender.

Prior to surrender, the subject will be fatigued and will have resigned himself to his fate. Some subjects may consider suicide more acceptable than surrender. The high expectations held hours before may have been dashed, leading to another failure on a long list of failures. The failure may be so great that long after the situation is over, the subject still will not move. The hostage taker sits dwelling on the greatest possible failure, when the venture was begun with the strong belief that triumph was possible.

Trained hostage negotiators understand that the subject is experiencing a great sense of loss and are able to assist the individual in surrendering with dignity. Further, they are aware of the differences between the rituals of surrender and rituals of suicide and are trained to react accordingly. Experienced law enforcement officers recognize that the subject may delay walking out the door into the custody of the law. While the hostage gains freedom, the subject is giving up one prison for another. The thinking negotiator gives the surrender an appearance of dignity in various ways, perhaps by allowing the hostage taker to carry out any money that was obtained or by allowing the individual to speak to the hostages afterward.

Suicide is a more likely solution for inadequate personality types than for any other type of hostage taker. The inadequate personality probably recognizes that he is in over his head and may be unwilling to face another failure. Suicide may occur to him as a positive solution, since he believes that anything is better than failing again. Suicide is also a method of getting even with others through passive-aggressive behavior.

A major problem with suicide in any hostage situation is the subject's inability to kill himself. The inadequate personality may see suicide as a reasonable solution, yet, because of his inability to pull the trigger, he could create a situation where the police must shoot him. This could occur in several ways. He could agree to surrender and then begin to shoot at the police. He could walk out with a hostage and then, at a critical moment, shoot at the hostage in order to force the police to shoot him. He could purposely disobey the instructions of the officer directing the surrender and thus force the police to shoot him.

Additionally, under the strain of the situation, the inadequate subject may talk to the negotiator about surrender, when he is actually planning suicide. While it is common, according to Bolz,[16] for a subject to want to shave, shower, change clothes, and make himself presentable before being taken into custody, other seemingly innocent activities may signal suicide. For example, a subject who tells the negotiator that he has been arrested previously and lost personal items in the process may be setting the stage for suicide. The subject may point out that when he was arrested, the jailer or arresting officer confiscated a watch and lost it. The subject may suggest that, to avoid such a problem and the embarrassment it may cause the police, the negotiator assist in disposing of any such items before surrender. He may begin to talk about giving possessions to various friends and family members. In fact, this type of discussion is a last will and testament. Bolz suggests thought interruption as an excellent ploy to alter the subject's line of conversation.[16]

Bolz recounts the story of one subject who stood on a roof eight stories above the pavement, holding his infant child over the edge, threatening to jump with him if he was not granted custody. The police told him that they would guarantee a day in family court in order to help him resolve the custody dispute. He agreed and told the police that he would come down off the ledge in just a few moments. However, before leaving the ledge he began to empty his pockets. Bolz recognized this as part of the suicide ritual, and, on that blistering August afternoon, asked the subject if he thought it would snow. The subject stopped everything, moved away from the ledge, and began to argue, saying, "You mean rain, not snow." The ploy was effective; Bolz then changed the topic and kept talking. The hostage taker calmed down, gave the baby to the police, and surrendered.[16]

Law Enforcement

Alarm

While uncontrolled emotions make the siege room atmosphere untenable for the subject, the situation is equally anxiety-provoking for the law enforcement officials. The officers who first responded were probably newer members of the department who were working their beat in a routine fashion. Like that of the hostages, their routine was dramatically broken.

In any situation like this, law enforcement officers may overreact, thinking that every person running from the siege site is a criminal about to shoot at civilians or at the police. Officers intend to expend every ounce of energy, risking their lives if necessary, to resolve, or at least contain, the incident.

Crisis

During the crisis stage, the forces outside the siege room are also fortifying their positions. A high level of professional action occurs. Various crowd control procedures are implemented and perimeters established. The patrol officer who was maintaining the inner perimeter is replaced by the sniper-observer team. The command post is established and early intelligence is gathered. The commander may learn who the subjects are, what their demands may be, and, most important, who the hostages are—primary victims of this crisis.

The initial intelligence is a combination of the most accurate and inaccurate information the police receive. For instance, during the Croatian takeover of the German Consulate in Chicago in August 1978, it was learned that there were two subjects and eight hostages. The hostages were correctly identified. However, early intelligence from a released hostage led law enforcement officials to believe that one of the subjects was on heroin. This was later found to be inaccurate. During this same stage of a siege in California, a white male hostage was able to take the weapon away from the white male subject. The hostage then ran from the building with the weapon. The police mistook him for the subject and shot him.[17]

Accommodation

By the time the accommodation phase sets in, Special Weapons and Tactics (SWAT) teams have been posted and sniper-observer teams have begun to report intelligence. The negotiator is in regular contact with the subject and reports observations to the commander. Detectives are gathering background data on the subject and the hostages. Officers have obtained building plans and maps of the area, as well as information on various community resources that can be used in the situation. The police, while inducing fatigue in the subject and hostages, are establishing schedules that will allow their personnel maximum rest during the quiet hours and ensure total alertness during times of tension. This schedule also helps alleviate the inevitable boredom the officers face.

Soon a tactical plan is well under way and only minor adjustments are necessary to maintain the calm professional posture the department has achieved. With officers in position, the commander sorts through reports from field units seeking information that may cause modification of the planned course of action. The staff is kept aware of current information on the disposition of the siege.

Resolution

Like those of the subject, the reactions of law enforcement officers during this stage will depend upon the nature of the settlement. If the subject surrenders, law enforcement officers will take him into custody. The SWAT team will take responsibility for the subject while other officers are charged with handling the hostages. For the police, the end will be quiet, almost anticlimactic. In those rare cases terminated by police assault, however, the final moments will be dramatic for those law enforcement officers involved in the assault. In either case, the end will be a well-rehearsed drill put into action by dedicated professionals whose primary objective is to preserve the lives of hostages.

Hostage Experience

Alarm

The alarm phase for unprepared, law-abiding citizens forced into a life and death situation is traumatic. Suddenly their worlds are turned around and they may experience near paralyzing fear.[18] In this stage, the victims move from routine existences into sudden and dramatic encounters with violence and possibly death. The police, from whom they expect help, seem to be doing nothing. The hostage feels let down. The situation seems unreal. Common feelings of omnipotence and invulnerability are quickly overcome by confusion and defenselessness.[18]

Many hostages seek immediate psychological refuge in the defense mechanism of denial of reality. According to Anna Freud, "When we find denial, we know that it is a reaction to external danger; when repression takes place, the ego is struggling with instinctual stimuli."[19]

In my interviews with hostages, they frequently discuss this use of denial of reality. According to McClure, the findings of denial are not limited to hostages:

> As I continued to talk to victims of violence, I became aware that the general reactions of these victims were similar to the psychological response of an individual who experiences sudden and unexpected loss. Loss of any kind, particularly if sudden and unexpected, produces a certain sequence of response in all individuals. The first response is shock and denial.[20]

Denial is a primitive but effective psychological defense mechanism that is put into use when the mind is so overloaded with trauma that it cannot handle the situation. Victims who cope effectively have strong wills to survive. Some may deal with the stress by believing that they are dreaming and will soon wake up. Some deal with the stress by sleeping—somnolent withdrawal. I have interviewed hostages who have slept for more than 90 percent of their time as captives. Some have fainted, although this is rare. In this context, it may be useful to understand panic, a hysterical and counterproductive reaction to stress. Panic occurs when the chances of a favorable outcome are perceived to diminish rapidly. In the event of a sudden shock, such as being taken hostage, people who have not been prepared may panic. Advance preparation can help potential victims avoid this extremely maladaptive response to the stress of becoming a hostage.[11]

Hostages have also repressed their fears. Frequently, fear of the hostage taker is transferred to a fear of the police. This is one element of the Stockholm Syndrome, which will be discussed later.

Crisis

The crisis phase is of critical importance to the survival of the hostage. The behavior pattern exhibited in this stage creates the precedent for hostage-subject interaction that can maximize the survival of the hostage. During the crisis phase, as in the alarm phase, some hostages still rely heavily on the defense mechanism of denial. Others are beginning to outgrow their denial and face reality. They begin to act as they do in normal circumstances. This behavior provides a measure of emotional relief and mental escape.

The stress individuals experience at this point may be due to their personal fears of isolation, claustrophobia, or the loss of their senses of time. Depending upon the length of captivity, these three psychological hazards may be very troublesome.

The first, isolation, can be particularly difficult for the more gregarious hostages. Such individuals must be able to handle both the demoralizing effect of being left totally alone and the fact that the only human contact they might have for extended periods of time will be with individuals who tend to be hostile.[10]

The second concern is claustrophobia. Darkness in a confined space for an extended period of time can be suffocating. Even in an aircraft of some size, space usually appears reduced because of terrorist (hijacker) demands that all window shades be pulled down. The terrorist may also require that all individuals remain in their seats with their seat belts fastened and tray tables down. Even the most sedentary individuals begin to feel the stress of such confinement. At the extreme are the individuals who are alone in their cells for months and cannot stand erect during their imprisonments. Sir Geoffrey Jackson, the British Ambassador to Uruguay, was taken hostage by the Tupamaros and held for 244 days. He spent three months in a cell measuring five by seven feet. Others have spent a similar amount of time in enclosures without windows, using a hole as a toilet, and one small light bulb as the only source of illumination. Hostages have survived such conditions.[10]

The third hazard experienced by hostages is the loss of a sense of time. The only knowledge hostages have of real time is that which their captors decide to relate. The knowledgeable hostage taker can effectively exploit this and enlist the assistance of the hostages against law enforcement. This manipulation has proven effective, as the Japanese Red Army and the South Moluccans learned during their sieges in 1977.

Accommodation

During the accommodation phase, the hours may seem like days to the captive. Boredom is broken only by moments of terror. This alternation of emotions induces fatigue.

Some hostages who survive develop what is now called the Stockholm Syndrome. One definition of the Stockholm Syndrome takes into account three phases of the experience and described it as:

> The positive feelings of the captives toward their captor(s) that are accompanied by negative feelings toward the police. These feelings are frequently reciprocated by the captor(s). To achieve a successful resolution of a hostage situation, law enforcement must encourage and tolerate the first two phases so as to induce the third and thus preserve the lives of all participants.[21]

The three phases, then, are (1) positive feelings on the part of the captives toward the captor; (2) negative feelings toward authorities on the part of the captives; and (3) positive feelings of the captor for the captives. This last step can spell the difference between life and death.

It appears that the Stockholm Syndrome is a coping device that most frequently is specific to the hostage. It is doubtful that the involvement is a conscious process in which the victim intends to manipulate the captor through personal identification. Reports indicate that victims who experience the Stockholm Syndrome try to resist their feelings of compassion for their captor.[21]

Some scientists consider identification with a captor a primitive attachment that stems from death imagery—a force about which little is known. It may be related to an individual's anticipation of death. A hostage is extremely vulnerable and might be expected to express attachment and even affection toward other persons present. On the whole, it may be difficult to feel compassion for a captor, particularly one whose behavior has been brutal; but, that captor may represent to the hostage the continued existence of authority and ability to deal with the situation. However, in certain group situations where a degree of interpersonal cohesiveness exists among the hostages, they may attend to one another's needs and not demonstrate reliance on the captors.[11]

If the positive feeling expressed by a hostage toward a captor is reciprocated, the victim will be better off. The outcome of an incident may be affected if the reciprocation occurs without manipulation—that is, if there is an unconscious genuineness to the relation. If a victim attempts to encourage a captor to feel some attachment, it would be important to allow the necessary feelings of natural warmth, empathy, and understanding to occur over time. Here again, the importance of the dictum "be yourself" is obvious.[11]

A moving account of this type of relationship is presented by Ochberg as he recounts the experience of one hostage of the South Moluccans in December 1975. Gerald Vaders, a newspaper editor in his fifties, told Ochberg the following:

> On the second night they tied me again to be a living shield and left me in that position for seven hours. The one who was most psychopathic kept telling me 'your time has come. Say your prayers.' They had selected me for the third execution. In the morning when I knew I was going to be executed, I asked to talk to Prins (another hostage) to give him a message to take to my family. I want to explain my family situation. My foster child, whose parents had been killed, did not get along too well with my wife, and I had at the time a crisis in my marriage just behind me. . . . There were other things too. Somewhere I had the feeling that I had failed as a human being. I explained all this and the terrorists insisted on listening.[22]

When Vaders completed his conversation with Prins and announced his readiness to die, the South Moluccans said, "No, someone else goes first."[22]

Ochberg observed that Vaders was no longer a faceless symbol. He was human. In the presence of executioners, he made the transition from a symbol to be executed to a human to be spared. The Moluccans selected another individual, Mr. Bierling, led him away, and executed him before they had the opportunity to know him.[22]

Vaders goes on to explain his experience of the Stockholm Syndrome:

> And you had to fight a certain feeling of compassion for the Moluccans. I know this is not natural, but in some way they come over human. They gave us cigarettes. They give us blankets. But we also realize that they were killers. You try to suppress that in your consciousness. And I knew I was suppressing that. I also knew that they were victims, too. In the long run they would be as much victims as we. Even more. You saw their morale crumbling. You experienced the disintegration of their personalities. The growing of despair. Things dripping through their fingers. You couldn't help but feel a certain pity. For people at the beginning with egos like gods—impregnable, invincible—they end up small, desperate, feeling that all was in vain.[22]

This affection for the aggressor occasionally arises in the protracted hostage situation. Perhaps dependence is a factor. The hostage is utterly helpless. When helplessness first occurred in infancy, it led to complete submission to the mother.[10] Perhaps this attraction to the hostage taker can be likened to the parent-child relationship.

Hostages often develop the idea that the police are the cause of their problems. It is common for hostages to tell themselves and each other that the siege would end if the police would go home.

Other hostages who survived and endured their ordeal with dignity have been known to gain strength by exploiting a perceived weakness of their captor. Though this behavior can be dangerous, successful exploitation can improve hostage morale. Marines in Tehran were threatened with immediate execution by their captors. They soon learned that this threat was a bluff and began to tell their captors where they wanted to be shot. They harassed their captors, as they had been harassed in boot camp. They exploited their captors' weaknesses. This behavior enabled them to improve their morale, make their captivity more tolerable, and survive without experiencing the Stockholm Syndrome.[14]

According to McClure, "Other arrogant hostages are Dr. Fly and Sir Geoffrey Jackson, who were so proud and influential that the terrorist organization found it necessary to remove the guards who were falling under their influence."[3] (Dr. Claude Fly was an American agronomist who was held by the Tupamaros for 208 days in 1970.)

However, most hostages are not individuals of the strength of character of Claude Fly, Geoffrey Jackson, or the captured Marines and cannot retain an air of aloofness during their captivities.

Resolution

Victim reaction during the final stage has been mixed; the physical reaction of the hostage is one of exhaustion. The depletion of energy required for resistance and retaining one's dignity becomes apparent. The moment of release may be greeted with vigor. However, chances are that the hostage's reservoir of energy has run out.

The hostages may have mixed feelings toward the subjects. Perhaps one of the most revealing descriptions of this inner conflict was offered by a stewardess who had been on the hijacked TWA flight 355:

> After it was over and we were safe, I recognized that they [the subjects] had put me through hell and had caused my parents and fiance a great deal of trauma. Yet, I was alive. I was alive because they had let me live. You know only a few people, if any, who hold your life in their hands and then give it back to you. After it was

over, and we were safe and they were in handcuffs, I walked over to them and kissed each one and said, "Thank you for giving me my life back." I know how foolish it sounds, but that is how I felt.[23]

This gratitude expressed by one stewardess reflects the feelings of hundreds of hostages. What she did not say is that her feelings toward her rescuers were less than gracious. Many former captives evidence hostility toward those who rescued them. Not only were the rescuing forces absent from the trauma within the siege room, they were assumed by hostages to have caused the trauma.

Although this confusion has been reflected in an attitude of gratitude toward the subjects for not hurting hostages, a fear exists that the hostage taker may escape from jail and take one hostage again.

Reports on former hostages suggest that a variety of physical and psychological problems may emerge long after the siege. Post-trauma anxiety may appear in the form of nightmares, nightsweats, startle reactions, and phobias. Some hostages were able to cope with some of these problems by not flying on a particular airline or avoiding the building in which they were held hostage.[24]

Ochberg reports finding in some hostages difficulties that range from mild depression to such serious psychological problems as survivor's guilt. A few have reported a form of paranoia reflected by a fear of future victimization by South American national terrorists striking in London.[25]

McClure has a more positive view of the fate of former hostages. He says that victims selected by terrorists, or those working in institutions selected for victimization, are usually people of recognized worth. They have accomplished something in their lives and probably have above-average qualities. When such people are properly prepared for the roles they may have to play as hostages, it is possible to improve their chances of surviving the experience with a minimum of aftereffects.[10]

William Niehous looks back upon his 40 months as a hostage in the jungles of Argentina with amazing strength. In an interview he said, "It is a hell of a way to quit smoking and lose weight. I was chained to a tree for 40 months, but I had a long chain."[26]

Recommendations for Survival

Alarm

Certain behavior is recommended during the alarm phase. The reaction to the first minutes of a hostage situation is best described by the American ambassador to Colombia, Diego Asencio: "The worst aspect of the ordeal was initial trauma. In the first few minutes, lie very close to the floor."[27] Asencio lived as a hostage for two months in the Dominican Embassy in Bogota. Although he later was to alter his behavior, his most enthusiastic advice to victims of any hostage situation is to disregard any notion of heroics or curiosity. Unarmed, untrained, and poorly conditioned civilians can best ensure survival by maintaining low profiles.

Crisis

During the crisis phase and all subsequent stages of the situation, individuals should remain conscious of their professional roles. Those without responsibilities for others may have the freedom to display their emotions; but this behavior may be dangerous if bothersome to the hostage takers. However, those with professional responsibilities for the safety of others cannot afford to vent their feelings. The trauma of a hospital-based hostage situation, a hijacking of commercial aircraft, the takeover of an embassy or an FBI office, or the aborted robbery of a bank casts many individuals into responsible roles.

One of our major airlines makes this role clear on each flight when the cabin attendants display the various safety equipment. They ask all passengers to pay attention to "the most important safety feature on the aircraft "— the crew.

When Sir Geoffrey Jackson was taken hostage, he remained in thought and actions the ambassador, the queen's representative. He so impressed his captors with his dignity that they were forced to change his guards regularly and isolate him for fear he might convince the guards that his cause was just and theirs foolish.[10]

Fly gained the respect of his captors and survived. He accomplished this by writing a 600-page autobiography and by developing a 50-page "Christian checklist" in which he analyzed the *New Testament*. Like Jackson, he was able to engage in comfortable, dignified behavior and insulate himself from the hostile pressures around him.[28]

Many individuals have survived hostage experiences by engaging in routine, dignified, nonthreatening behavior. This is a common tactic of stewardesses or pilots on commercial aircraft. Those who survive tend to busy themselves during the siege with their professional responsibilities. They tend to take refuge in normal behavior, which enables them and their passengers to survive the ordeal.[24]

For example, on an otherwise quiet Sunday afternoon in late June 1981, a white male outpatient who had been previously diagnosed as a paranoid schizophrenic took hostages in a southeastern law enforcement agency. The siege lasted for several hours. During the course of negotiations, the switchboard operator remained at her station and handled calls as she had been trained. She appeared to find refuge and comfort in the familiar, nonthreatening routine. In subsequent interviews of the hostages, FBI agents and psychiatrists verified that the switchboard operator survived with the least amount of trauma.[29]

Even though comfortable, routine, dignified behavior has enabled many members of flight crews to survive, this type of behavior can create problems when it threatens the subject. When Captain Schuman, the pilot of Lufthansa 181, was hijacked by four members of the Palestine Liberation Organization (PLO) in the fall of 1977, his interpretation of appropriate behavior was fatal. As the pilot, Schuman considered himself in command of the aircraft. However, the lead terrorist, Zuhair Mousot Akkash, who called himself Captain Mahmoud, was intimidated by Captain Schuman's behavior. Akkash could have been an inadequate personality who took the title of captain as compensation for his feelings of inferiority. Captain Schuman may have sensed and exploited this inadequacy. Since Akkash had a weapon and could not tolerate the competition from the real captain of the aircraft, he executed Schuman at Dubai.

Diego Asencio advises, "Try to maintain your dignity and don't become too passive."[30] Thus, the activity of hostages to ensure survival seems relatively simple. They must retain their dignity without antagonizing their captors.

To some extent, stamina and the ability to absorb physical punishment, or, more accurately, endure poor food and cramped conditions, is important. Yet some who have survived with dignity have been elderly individuals with health problems. A philosophical disposition and emotional stability may be more important survival factors than physical conditioning.[31]

Dr. Claude Fly credited his survival to his spiritual strength. More common personality traits that also increase the chance of survival are patience, a sense of humor, sympathy, self-control, and objectivity.

Panic, crying, and verbal assault of the captors are certainly as likely to spell an early demise as dignity, an ability to laugh at oneself, and self-control are to enable one to survive.

Exploitation of subjects is not uncommon. The marine security guards held in Iran became aware of their captors' fear of them and successfully manipulated their captors to obtain favors and news of the world.[14]

A stewardess on Continental 72, which was commandeered at the terminal in Los Angeles in March 1981, served the subject, acted as his messenger, and performed other routine, nonthreatening tasks for him. As the hijacking progressed from 10 a.m. until almost 9 p.m., she encouraged him to release hostages. Eventually, she was the only hostage on board. When she perceived the time was right, she told the subject it was time for her to leave. She exited the aircraft and the subject surrendered.[32]

During this and each phase of the siege, hostages are cautioned not to do anything precipitous. Adaptation requires hostages to resist some basic drives. This marks the height of readiness with the organism on "high gain," prepared for total expenditure of energy.[11] Some hostages are given to verbal combat with their captors. This verbal interaction may include attempts to humiliate the subject. The concept of humiliation is very important in the precipitation of violence. Hostages should avoid confrontation or the temptation to humiliate the subject. Success in verbal combat may force the subject to act to save face.[33] This face saving has included the killing of a hostage. An example of this was when the articulate, outspoken Khomeini supporter, Abbas Lavasani, was held hostage in the Iranian Embassy in London in early 1980. His captors were less articulate Arabs from Khuzistan who could not counter his arguments and took exception to his arrogance. Lavasani was murdered by the terrorists while he was tied to the railing; his body was thrown from the embassy on the sixth day.[34]

During the hijacking of TWA 355 by a group of Croatians led by Zuvonko Busich, one hostage was abused. When other hostages were advised of this, they replied that he had it coming to him. He was acting like a baby, crying about a stomachache and irritating everyone.[35] This indicates that behavior that tends to draw attention to the hostage can be counterproductive, if not fatal.

During the early phase of the first Moluccan train siege in December 1975, Vaders had begun engaging in behavior that was typical of a newspaper editor. He kept a diary. This behavior distinguished him from the other hostages who were sitting and staring. The Moluccans took exception to Vaders' activity and singled him out. Terrorists do not like people who act too differently from the other hostages, regardless of how adaptive this behavior might seem.[36]

A common and effective activity is physical exercise. Most accounts of effective adaptive behavior discuss the importance of exercise and physical fitness.[37,38,39] Flexibility exercises are essential to minimize the risk of joint dislocations or bone fractures should the captors resort to physical abuse.[40] Running in place promotes endurance, cardiovascular fitness, and more sound sleep patterns. Additionally, such activity helps the hostage cope with boredom and enables the individual to gain the sense of accomplishing something worthwhile during this period.

Accommodation

The recommended behavior for the accommodation phase is similar to that described for the crisis phase. The research of the Rand Corporation was quoted earlier to support the statement that most hostages are injured or die early in a siege as the transition is made from the failed robbery to the hostage situation or when an assault is called for to terminate the negotiation stalemate. Therefore, the hostage who has survived through the accommodation phase must be doing something right. By this stage, most hostages understand their captors and know how to manipulate them to remain alive. Therefore, the recommended behavior for this phase is to continue the behavior that has sustained each hostage through the second phase.

Resolution

By the termination phase—hours or days by the clock, but years of emotional time—most hostages will have little difficulty doing what they are told. However, when the siege ends, hostages must follow the instructions of law enforcement officials.

Should the ordeal be terminated by assault, an entirely different course of action is dictated as compared to that recommended in a situation resolved by the surrender of the subjects. A violent end to a hostage situation is not a pleasant experience for anyone. The moment an assault is launched, hostages are encouraged to lie on the floor. In the event of an aircraft hijacking, they should assume the crash landing position in their seats. In any case, hostages should keep their hands in clear sight by interlacing their fingers over their heads. They should expect more terror during resolution than during the crisis phase, heightened by the smell of tear gas and its effects, smoke from fires, and shooting and yelling.

The rescuing forces will have practiced their assault plans perhaps a hundred times. Their mission is to neutralize the subjects and protect all hostages from harm. The terror created by the noise and rapid movement of the rescuing forces is intended to induce a state of confusion in the subjects. The hostages, however, are subject to a similar reaction. Therefore, they should remain very still. Precipitous movement by a hostage during these moments of confusion could be considered a hostile act by the rescuing forces. When these forces want hostages to move, they will instruct them to do so with clear and concise orders. In some instances, the forces will move hostages.

A peaceful surrender is preferred and is the most common end in sieges. The FBI has terminated less than a dozen of more than 250 hijackings in shootings. In a quiet surrender of the subjects, the hostages will have an easier time following the instructions of law enforcement officials. There have been situations in which the subjects have tried to filter out of the siege site with their hostages. Therefore, until a formal identification has been completed, hostages should expect to be searched and treated as if they were subjects. This treatment may include handcuffing and will include careful monitoring of hostage behavior until identification is certain.

In either situation, hostages should also expect to be detained by rescuing forces for interviews to gather evidence for a future appearance in court. Medical and psychiatric procedures may also be in order before hostages are reunited with their families and friends.

EPILOGUE

Writers on hostage recovery are united in their concern for the mental health of former hostages. McClure, Jenkins, and Ochberg all recommend that former hostages and their families consider some professional help to get them through the post-release experience. One excellent course of information for those who may be called upon to treat former hostages is the article by Rahe and Genender entitled "Adaption to and Recovery from Captivity Stress."[18] It points out that a major treatment problem is that, while in captivity, hostages survive by becoming self-reliant, while effective use of therapy may require reliance on others. Some former hostages experience difficulty in making this shift.[18] Dr. Reid adds that the therapist should be consistent, allow full ventilation prior to any specific therapy, and consider leaving simple symptoms alone unless the patient finds them particularly distressing.[37]

Few can understand the emotions of former hostages. Try as we may, we can only provide sympathy; another former hostage can provide the empathy that seems necessary. Many hostages have undergone profound religious experiences, or at least a deepening of religious faith. They return to their families and friends as new people. This requires some adjustment for everyone involved. Some hostages report guilt feelings. They say that they feel it was somehow their own fault that they were taken.

Family and friends can be most helpful by allowing the former hostage to tell the story, to ventilate. Hostages should be allowed and enabled to survive this trauma with the dignity they demonstrated while captive. As Niehous said, "Without survival, there is no victory."[26]

"The bottom line," according to Frank Ochberg, "is that no concise formula for survival exists. However, one can help ensure his safety through awareness, being mature and possessing some luck."[41]

This paper has focused upon the first of Dr. Ochberg's tenets, the importance of information on what to expect. Information is also the basis of the first phase of crisis intervention. Improved self-awareness will grow from reflection upon how individuals think they might behave under such stress. Maturity is a matter of personal growth, and information should contribute to such development. I believe one makes luck; thoughtful preparation for victimization is a way of doing just that.

NOTES

1. Daniel Lang, "Reporter at Large," *New Yorker*, November 1974, p. 56.

2. Brian M. Jenkins, Janera Johnson, and David Ronfeldt, *Numbered Lives: Some Statistical Observations from Seventy-Seven International Hostage Episodes* (Santa Monica, Ca: Rand Corporation, 1977).

3. U. S. Congress, Senate Committee on the Judiciary, *Terrorist Activity; Hostage Defense Measures, Hearings before a subcommittee to investigate the administration of the Internal Security Act and other security laws*, Part 5, 94th Cong., 1st Sess., 1975.

4. F. M. Ochberg, "The Victim of Terrorism: Psychiatric Considerations," *Terrorism: An International Journal* 1 (1978): 2.

5. J. D. Moore, "Spokane's Robbery Education Program," *FBI Law Enforcement Bulletin* 49 (1980): 11.

6. Interview of Arish R. Turle, Vice President, Control Risks Limited, Miami Beach, Florida, February 18, 1981.

7. B. Graves and T. Strentz, "The Kidnaper: His Crime and His Background," research paper (Special Operations and Research Staff, FBI Academy, Quantico, Virginia, 1977), p. 20

8. S. M. Auerbach and P. R. Kilmann, "Crisis Intervention: A Review of Outcome Research," *Psychological Bulletin* 84 (1977): 1189-1217.

9. F. M. Ochberg, Address to the Third International Terrorist Symposium, FBI Academy, June 26, 1980, Quantico, Virginia.

10. B. McClure, "Hostage Survival," in *International Terrorism in the Contemporary World* , eds. M. H. Livingston, L. B. Kress, and M.G. Wanek (Westport: Greenwood Press, 1978), p. 281.

11. F. M. Ochberg, "Preparing for Terrorist Victimization," in *Political Terrorism and Business* , eds. Y. Alexander and R. Kilmark (New York: Praeger Special Studies, 1979), p. 118.

12. Interview of Dr. Charles Russel, FBI Academy, June 25, 1980.

13. N.R.F. Maier, "Assets and Liabilities in Group Problem Solving: The Need for an Integrative Function," in *Classics of Organization Behavior*, ed. W.E. Natemeyer (Oak Park, Ill: Moore Publishing Company, 1978), p. 140.

14. Interviews with U.S. Marine security guards who were hostages in various cities in Iran for 444 days, Quantico, Virginia, March, 1981.

15. Dr. Harley Stock, Ph.D., Lecture to hostage negotiators at FBI Academy, Quantico, Virginia, April 1981.

16. F. Bolz and E. Hershey, *Hostage Cop* (New York: Rawson Wade, 1979), p. 57.

17. Francis Bolz, Address to the Third International Terrorist Symposium, FBI Academy, Quantico, Virginia, June 1980.

18. Richard H. Rahe and E. Genender, "Adaptation to and Recovery from Captivity Stress," *Military Medicine* 148 (1983): 577-585.

19. A. Freud, *The Ego and the Mechanisms of Defense*, rev. ed. (New York: International Universities Press, 1974), p. 109.

20. B. McClure, "Hostage Survival," Preliminary draft of research findings, 1978, pp. 17-18.

21. T. Strentz, "The Stockholm Syndrome: Law Enforcement Policy and Ego Defenses of the Hostage," *The Law Enforcement Bulletin*, April 1979, pp. 1-11.

22. F. M. Ochberg, "The Victims of Terrorism: Psychiatric Considerations," *Terrorism* 1 (1977): 147-168.

23. Interviews with Ms. Kathy Robinson, Stewardess on TWA 355, New York City, September 20, 1976.

24. Interviews with Flight Deck Crew and Stewardess on TWA 355, Washington, D. C. and New York City, October 1976; Interviews with victims of J.A.L. 472, Los Angeles, October 1977; and Interviews with the Malaysian Air Line crew that transported the Japanese Red Army Terrorists from Kuala Lumpur to Algeria, Kuala Lumpur, Malaysia, September 1979.

25. Interview with Sir Geoffrey Jackson, Hendon Hall at Scotland Yard Hostage Negotiators School, London, England, September 6, 1980.

26. Interview with Mr. William F. Niehous, Toledo, Ohio, October 24, 1979.

27. "Honor Awarded Hostage Envoy," *Washington Star*, April 12, 1980.

28. C. L. Fly, *No Hope But God* (New York: Hawthorn, 1973), pp. 115-220.

29. C. L. Wesslius. and J. V. DeSarno, Jr., "The Anatomy of a Hostage Situation," *Behavioral Sciences and the Law* 1, no. 2 (1983): 33-46.

30. "Honor Awarded Hostage Envoy," *Washington Star*, April 12, 1980.

31. J. B. Stockdale, "World Epictitus Reflection on Survival and Leadership," *Atlantic*, April 1978, pp. 98-106.

32. Interview with Ms. Barbara Sorenson, in Los Angeles, California, March 1981.

33. Personal communication from Dr. William H. Reid, M. D., MPH, Associate of Psychiatry, University of Nebraska Medical Center, Omaha, Nebraska, May 9, 1983.

34. Personal communication from Detective Superintendent David Veness, New Scotland Yard, London SWI England, July 1983.

35. Interview of Victims of TWA Flight 355 in New York City, October 1976.

36. Ochberg, "The Victims of Terrorism: Psychiatric Considerations," p. 151.

37. John G. Hubbell, *P. O. W.,* The Readers Digest Press, 1976.

38. L. M. Bucher, *Bucher: My Story.* Garden City, New York: Doubleday, 1970.

39. E. R. Murphy, *Second in Command*, New York: Holt, Rinehart, and Winston, 1971.

40. J. E. Nardini, "Psychiatric Concepts of Prisoners of War Confinement," *Military Medicine* 127 (1952): 229-307.

41. Personal Communication from Dr. Frank M. Ochberg, M.D., September 3, 1982.

Chapter 12

Security Management for Health Care Administrators

Wade Ishimoto

OVERVIEW

This chapter represents a departure from traditional security approaches, as it presents eclectic courses of action for consideration by administrators and medical security planners. The rationale for this approach is that, while the principles of security may remain constant, the manner in which those principles are applied will differ because of great variances in individual circumstances and setting. The authors believe that specific security practices, hospital-wide training, and systems must be individualized to meet an institution's needs in a cost-effective and secure manner.

INTRODUCTION

How do you view security? This simple question evokes a variety of responses from administrators, medical staff members, security professionals, and patients. Their responses range from apathy to a firm commitment to effective security. Differing views on security are understandable and must be considered in planning and managing security matters. Of course, it is ludicrous to adopt procedures that try to satisfy each and every perception and to believe that a particular procedure will be the panacea for every potential security problem. Please take careful note of the word "perception." Perception, indeed, does play an important role in security management and will reappear throughout this chapter.

Obviously, you are concerned about violence in health care settings. Perhaps your concerns and your approaches to security are not the same as those of others. However, if you are involved in the management of security for your institution, such differences must be settled in a manner that ultimately will provide cost-effective security. This chapter will address methods for determining how to plan, organize, and manage the security function.

ANALYSIS

In emergency situations, medical practitioners are often faced with treating their patients symptomatically and in such a way that full analysis is not possible because of time or other constraints. If you are presently in an emergency security situation, this chapter will be of little benefit to you. Let us assume, however, that you do have the time to do detailed analysis for security purposes. The time you spend on this analysis and in reading this chapter should pay long-term dividends both in preventing incidents, and, in the event that an incident does occur, in replacing an uncoordinated reaction with a timely and orderly response. This analysis will also allow those that are involved in the security planning and decision-making process to agree on perceptual matters before dollars are wasted.

In many ways, security is a matter of perception and becomes a highly emotional issue at times. While no one can claim that all emotion can be divorced from security planning decisions or that all differences in opinion or program emphasis can be settled, the introduction of a logical, analytical process at least should decrease the emotion that often becomes a disruptive factor in security planning.

Persons in the security industry have coined a number of different descriptive (and nondescriptive) names for the analysis you are about to perform. You will hear such terms as surveys, assessments, vulnerability analyses, and risk analyses. The names should be of little concern to you, for your main interest is to get the job done. The critical point, then, is determining what should be contained in this analysis.

Table 12-1 suggests a basic framework for your analysis. Each of the different parts will be explained in greater detail in the remainder of the chapter. The end result of your analysis will be the capability to structure plans and programs to meet your specific needs, to organize your security efforts, and to implement security operations.

The outline provided in Table 12-1 also may be used as a format for recording the results of your analysis. Formal written recording of the analysis is well worth the effort, since the record can serve as a primer for those new employees that will have vital roles in security matters, become a basis for future review, and provide justification for budgetary matters.

Table 12-1 Framework for Analysis

Institutional goals, functions, and operations
Institutional organization
People-oriented security priorities
The institutional setting: the geographical setting, image
  considerations, and limitations
The threat
The vulnerabilities to the threat
Total risk assessment
Evaluation of existing security and safety

Institutional Goals, Functions, and Operations

What is the value of recording and analyzing this information? Security must support the institution. All too often, individuals believe that security exists for its own sake and that the institution should support security. By stating what your institution must do to stay in operation, you indirectly will have stated how security can enhance that ability to operate.

The goals of the institution may also be called its mission. Since there is no medical institution that can realistically provide health care to everyone, any time, any place, you will find some limiting factors in the goal or mission statements that will aid in defining the security function. For example, the goal for Hospital X may be to provide general inpatient and emergency care under one roof on a continual basis for upper income persons principally residing in Area Y. An analysis for security purposes would then indicate that security may have to be provided 24 hours a day, that security personnel will have to be able to relate to the perceptions and requests of upper income persons, and that there is only one physical location that you must be concerned with securing.

Whereas the goals provide an overview, an analysis of the institution's exact functions and methods of operation will provide an in-depth view of what kind of security may be required, and where and when it will be needed. These must be carefully documented and recorded. Pay particular attention to those functions and operations that are critical to the fulfillment of the institution's mission. Those are apt to be the areas in which security is needed. Pay particular attention to the support and administrative areas, because they may require more attention than some of the purely medical areas. As an example, any funds stored in the building require some type of protection.

Organization

The first step designates what the institution must do to accomplish its goals. The second step provides a view of how the institution is organized to meet those goals. How does that help to manage security? One of the many things it does is to identify key personnel that should be involved in security matters. These key persons may be used to determine the impact of security programs and also as extensions of the security force. No security or law enforcement organization can exist without the help of those they are trying to protect.

A closer look at organization reveals other useful information for security planning. You will be able to see the flow of funds, drugs, and other items that will probably require some type of protection. You will see patterns of pedestrian and vehicular traffic flow. You will know where certain sensitive information and equipment are located and how they are maintained. Your review of organization, combined with the review of goals, functions, and operational methods, should give you much information concerning what must be safeguarded.

Persons to Safeguard

The next step you might take is to determine who must be safeguarded.

Your analysis should begin with a clear understanding of what categories of personnel your institution has the responsibility to safeguard. The 1983 *Accreditation Manual for Hospitals*[1] states, "Security measures will be taken to provide security for patients, personnel, and the public. . . ." These three general categories of persons may be further broken down to meet your particular needs, as illustrated in Table 12-2.

Table 12-2 is a sample listing. You may choose to expand the list based on your particular situation. For example, the establishment of identification procedures that limit access to certain areas may require you to subdivide medical staff personnel into residents, interns, and nurses.

The main objective in categorizing persons is to assist you in determining specific security procedures that will be required to safeguard different categories of persons. A secondary objective is to help you in realizing what perceptions must be either considered or projected in your development of security programs and measures. The medical institution's public image is an important consideration that has an impact on the institution's ability to operate, and, therefore, affects security matters.

Table 12-2 Persons to Safeguard

> PATIENTS
> Ambulatory
> Nonambulatory
> Prisoners
> Mental patients
>
> PERSONNEL
> Medical staff
> Support staff
> Utility and maintenance staff
> Vendors
> Volunteers
>
> PUBLIC
> Visitors
> Neighbors

The Environmental Impact

You have obtained a good idea of who and what to protect. You should now look at where this protection is needed. You obtained some information concerning the *where* during your first two steps of this analysis. However, you must now attend to three additional considerations: (1) the physical setting; (2) weather; and (3) image.

Consideration of the physical setting requires information on terrain, boundaries, flora, fauna, and other factors that will have an important impact on how you secure the facility. Analysis of these factors will be vital in determining what specific items of security equipment are best for your facility and how you can integrate equipment with personnel to obtain a cost-effective solution for potential security problems.

Weather information includes data on temperature extremes, precipitation, and the probability of weather-related hazards in your area. Analysis of weather information will assist you in selecting items of security equipment, measuring the effects of weather on people, and in the development of integrated programs for security.

Image considerations are difficult to thoroughly address in a short treatise. Naturally, most medical institutions do not wish to project the appearance of an armed camp because of its adverse impact on neighbors, visitors, patients, and institutional personnel. That's easy to state; however, whether or not security guards should be uniformed and armed may not be so easy to determine. Knowing that you cannot please everyone is of little consolation, for a decision must still be made on which perceptions of the health care facility by which category of persons are most important. That image consciousness will probably lead to compromises in security measures, and the security planner must be adept and flexible in reaching compromises that will not unduly detract from the security mission.

Other Limitations

With your security analysis, you are determining limitations on how security will be accomplished. The nature of security is such that perfect, fail-safe security is impossible, so an elimination process becomes necessary.

Your research should consider the so-called compliance legislation and other de facto matters that have an impact on your security operations. You must consider such items as fire codes, medical institution accreditation standards, building codes, labor union agreements, Occupational Safety and Health Act (OSHA) standards, and budgetary restrictions.

Upon completing this step, you will know what you must do (compliance) and what you cannot do (limitation).

Threat, Vulnerabilities, and Risk

The next step is to determine why security is needed. This is really a matter of determining the threat to your particular institution and the persons connected with the institution. Threat is a strong word, but it is nonetheless a fact of life. Threat equals danger, and danger may come from natural or man-made events.

Do not, therefore, equate threat only with deliberately caused acts of violence carried out by people. People may inadvertently cause severe accidents that endanger others. People also steal, and unabated theft will certainly threaten the institution's ability to remain in operation. Mother nature also poses threats to your existence through hurricanes, storms, and earthquakes. Table 12-3 lists some potential threats of possible concern to you.

Table 12-3 is voluminous, but is not necessarily all-encompassing. Additions and deletions may be made depending on whether your viewpoint emphasizes protection or law enforcement. A variety of preventive measures will provide protection against the various forms of theft (e.g., burglary, larceny, pilferage, and shoplifting). The option you select will often be determined by legal considerations or local law enforcement practices. The latter will influence specific security procedures, report writing, and other measures. In the same vein, Table 12-3 treats terrorism under the particular

Table 12-3 Potential Threats

Natural Violence

Cyclones/Tornados/Typhoons/Wind	Snow and ice
Earthquakes	Structural collapse
Fire	Tidal waves
Flooding	
Hurricanes	

Man-Made Violence

Arson	Kidnapping
Assaults against facility	Murder and Manslaughter
Assaults against employees	Riots
Bombings	Robbery
Demonstrations	Sabotage
Disorderly conduct	Sex offenses
Drug offenses	Traffic accidents
Extortion	Violent accidents
Hijacking	

Nonviolent Man-Made Threats

Bad checks	Larceny
Burglary	Pilferage
Embezzlement	Shoplifting
Espionage	Theft
Forgery	Trespassing
Fraud	Unfair competition
Gambling	Vandalism

type of action or crime that it may cause, for example, murder, hijacking, and extortion.

To list the threats without determining their true impact on your institution would be meaningless. You must further analyze existing information to rate the degree of the specific threat against your institution. Probabilities of occurrence must be estimated, and these estimates must be reviewed periodically to see if any changes in priority are required.

While you engage in this process, you should also determine the institution's vulnerability against specific threats. This is one of the most important steps in your analytical process, for it will lead to a determination of costs. You determine vulnerabilities by retrieving the information you compiled previously on the institution's history, functions, operations, and organization. On one hand, you will be looking at what kind of target you may present or be perceived as presenting to criminals. On the other hand, you will be looking at what criminal activities traditionally have taken place at your type of facility or institution.

At this point, it would behoove you to determine what the postulated risks are in a weighted formula. Walsh and Healy, in *Protection of Assets Manual,*[2] list two formulas. One deals with loss event probability and the other with loss event criticality.

Loss event probability is stated by them as $P = f/n$ where

P = the probability that a given event will occur;

f = the number of outcomes or results favorable to the occurrence of the event; and

n = the total number of equally possible outcomes or results.

Walsh and Healy introduce a cost-of-loss formula as an intermediate step that is expressed as

$K = (C_p + C_t + C_r + C_d - (I - a)$ where

K = criticality

C_p = cost of permanent replacement

C_t = cost of temporary replacement

C_r = total related costs

C_d = discounted cash cost

I = available insurance or indemnity

a = allocable insurance premium amount

Loss event criticality is then listed by Walsh and Healy in five categorical ratings:

1 = fatal to the business

2 = very serious

3 = moderately serious

4 = relatively unimportant

5 = seriousness unknown

A simpler formula to determine criticality of loss is presented by Green and Farber in *Introduction to Security*[3] where

$ cost of each potential loss

x frequency of loss per year

= $ annual cost of loss

No matter what formula you use, you will take a major step in determining how you will provide cost-effective security for your institution. You also will arm yourself with cost figures that will be more understandable to other administrators and you will gain a means for evaluating security department budget requests. The end result is that you will have a very good idea of what needs protection and how those needs may best be met.

What Exists Now

The final step in your survey and analysis concerns what security programs, measures, personnel, and equipment are already in place. The administrators and you will gain a means for evaluating security department budget requests. The end result is that you will have a very good idea of what needs protection and how those needs may best be met.

What Exists Now

The final step in your survey and analysis concerns what security programs, measures, personnel, and equipment are already in place. The analysis should be oriented toward an evaluation of the cost-effectiveness in preventing and responding to viable security threats.

Precise checklists are beyond the scope of this chapter; however, you may find them in a variety of reference sources, such as the aforementioned *Protection of Assets Manual*[2] by Walsh and Healy. Of course, this does not tell you what you should survey. The following general areas should serve as a guideline:

1. Physical Security: Look at the types, locations, reliability, and effectiveness of barriers, lighting, locks and keys, closed circuit televisions, signs, and intrusion detection systems.[4]
2. Personnel Security: Review employee screening procedures, issuance and use of identification, access control measures, visitor control procedures, and designation of any restricted areas.
3. Package and Property Control: Measure what property exists to prevent theft and security hazards through inventory controls, movement restrictions, and screening. Also, examine your procedures for controlling drugs and controlled substances, including irradiated materials.
4. Information Security: Determine what measures exist to protect patient information, research data, and other sensitive institutional information. Proper protection also implies destruction measures.
5. Funds Security: This area includes measures to protect cash, valuables, and negotiable instruments.
6. Fire Protection: Consider detection and alarm equipment, fire-fighting equipment, the ability to use such equipment, and the existence of fire hazards.
7. Security Force Operations: Look at the responsibilities of the security forces and their adequacy to accomplish them. Review guard orders, plans, and contracts. Examine equipment, training, morale, and management procedures.
8. Emergency/Contingency/Crisis Plans: Determine what issues these plans address and how well they address those issues. When have they been tested?

9. Security Education Programs: Consider programs for security personnel and other employees.
10. Power Supply and Communications: Pay special attention to emergency power and communications systems, including maintenance, periodic inspection and testing, and the availability of supplies to keep them operating.
11. Occupational Safety and Health Act Requirements and Programs: Determine what measures are necessary to meet these requirements.

Determination

Your data collection and analysis should be just about finished at this stage. Perhaps you are breathing a sigh of relief or are buried in facts and figures. Nonetheless, your perseverance and determination will cause you to take a deep breath and plunge ahead.

Next, you must meticulously plan the operation of the security apparatus and gain approval for your plan. A likely first step is to determine and list exactly what security functions should and will be undertaken. Those functions may be subdivided into four major categories: (1) prevention; (2) detection; (3) response; and (4) security education. These four categories form the cornerstone of your security structure.

Intuitively, you know that it would be highly desirable to prevent all crimes and dangerous acts from occurring. However, the likelihood of preventing all incidents is virtually nil. Therefore, you must devise ways to detect and respond to these events. Finally, you can use security education to extend your security capabilities to others in order to multiply your protection.

Specific items of equipment and personnel should also be able to perform a variety of cross-category functions whenever possible. For instance, capable security guards act to prevent threats through their presence in particular locations. They may also detect crimes or dangerous situations before or as they are occurring, respond to events, and educate others on their responsibilities. Similarly, an intrusion detection system detects certain events and then aids response by triggering an alarm.

Clearly state your objectives within each of the four categories of security functions. Force yourself to be specific and refer back to the wealth of information you have already gathered. The principal question to ask yourself is, "Does this objective support the criticality ratings that were previously determined?" If the answer is no, you are probably wasting resources.

Once your objectives are stated and reviewed against the postulations that were formed in your risk analysis, list options that might meet your objectives. A spread sheet format is ideal for this process because your next two columns should list estimated annual costs for the options and appropriate comments. Table 12-4 illustrates this process.

This is a painstaking process. However, you will save money and other resources in the end. Should you decide not to perform this analysis, there will be little substance to your security planning. Instead of planning for security, you will find yourself reacting in a knee-jerk fashion to different situations. Instead of presenting adequate, coherent training to nurses, physicians, and others, you may present an unwanted and poorly directed program on the management of violent and disruptive behavior.

Table 12-4 Options

Objectives	Options	Estimated Annual Cost	Comments
(Clearly state your objectives.)	(Briefly explain the security measures that will support your objectives.)		(Enter applicable comments, for example, those that show why an option is favored.)
1. To prevent theft, assaults, and accidents in parking lot	1. Install increased lighting	+$10,000	1(a.) Costs include installation, operations, and maintenance 1(b.) Current lighting inadequate
	2. Assign foot patrol to randomly check lot once an hour	$0	2(a.) Added duty 2(b.) Permanent assignment to lot not deemed effective
	3. Trim shrubbery in northeast area of lot	$1,500	3(a.) In four incidents last year, suspects hid in area 3(b.) area is also an eyesore
	4. Request more patrolling by Police Dept.	?	4(a.) Police Dept. has $ shortage 4(b.) Off-duty officer for 8 hrs/day = $22k annually 4(c.) Option 2 is better

Before leaving this section on determining your objectives, options, and costs, list objectives and options that are already in operation and considered adequate for now. Doing so will assist you in budgetary projections and periodic reviews at a later date. If you are considering construction or structural modification of a facility, get someone involved in the planning process to consider security implications at an early time. This, again, is a cost-effective approach, since any wiring for security is much less expensive when undertaken during, rather than after, construction.

Organization/Reorganization for Security

Perhaps all of your work to date has shown the need to reorganize your security effort (or to organize it if you are planning to open a new facility). Three tasks will soon become necessary: (1) selecting a security director; (2) selecting other security personnel; and (3) selecting equipment.

Before you can select a security director, you must be able to clearly state what is expected from that person. You should state the functions, authority, and responsibilities, along with the salary and benefits you are willing to offer. The latter need not be stated outright to the interviewee, since you may wish to negotiate the exact figures, but you should be able to indicate a salary range.

By stating functions, authority, and responsibilities you will have established criteria for the selection of the security director. Those items, along with the compensation package, will steer you in your recruitment, interview, and selection process. It would be senseless for anyone outside your organization to establish selection criteria. This is your security director, and the person selected must meet your individualized needs and be compatible within your organization. By defining your criteria, you will be able to determine what type of person you need. Management talent hunters and certain security firms may aid you in your search for a security director, but you must participate in the interview process and in the ultimate decision. The security director need not automatically come from the ranks of law enforcement, military, intelligence, or security personnel. You may find that the director's principal duties will demand someone with a strong background in personnel management. In this case, your criteria should call for someone with that background who is trainable in security matters, or vice versa. Don't waste the hard work you have done in analyzing your security needs by hiring someone who cannot meet your criteria for security director. You won't be doing a favor for yourself or for the person you hired.

No matter whom you select as security director, one individual can't do it alone. Your particular situation and needs will determine how you augment and assist the security director in fulfilling the responsibilities. There are several major options:

- Rely on other employees who have other principal responsibilities.
- Use consultants to augment the efforts of the security director.
- Hire a small number of assistants for the director and rely on them as well as on other non-security employees.
- Hire off-duty law enforcement officers.
- Form a proprietary security guard force.
- Obtain contract security guard services.

There is no single correct solution. Your previous analysis will once more pay dividends in helping you make the correct decision for your institution and its specific needs. Additional factors to consider prior to making your decision include cost; ability to fulfill needs and objectives; reliability; image; personnel turbulence; and labor relations.

So much for the people side of security. People alone cannot provide adequate security in any but the most primitive of societies. Just as you need to augment the efforts of the security director with people, you must augment the human effort with equipment. A quick look at the selection of security equipment and a few do's and don't's follow. Do integrate persons and equipment in your plans. Don't rely totally on technology. Do state your requirements to bidders. Do look at maintenance and servicing prior to buying. Do consider leasing. Don't overbuy.

All too often, organizations buy excellent equipment that is absolutely wrong for their intended application. This is compounded by the failure to properly plan and contract or budget for servicing and maintenance, which often results in wasted monies and ineffective equipment. You can avoid these pitfalls through thorough planning and analysis of your requirements.

Plans

You are to be complimented if you have come this far. The analysis has been completed, the personnel have been hired, the security effort has been organized, and the equipment is in place. Before you rest on your laurels, have you prepared plans to specify how the security functions will be executed?

What kind of plans need to be prepared? What are the priorities? The answer to the first question is plans that deal with the four categories of security functions delineated earlier: (1) prevention; (2) detection; (3) response; and (4) security education.

Prevention plans include individual or integrated plans that deal with such areas as lock and key control, security of funds, and security of drugs. They may be so detailed as to include individual guard orders. To preclude unnecessary duplication, these plans, where possible, should include matters pertaining to detection, response, and applicable education.

Detection plans should be capable of being addressed in such items as a Patrol Plan. Other means of detection like inventories, audits, and inspections may again be included under separate prevention plans such as a Drug Security Plan. A maintenance, test, and servicing plan for your intrusion detection system would probably best be addressed in an overall Physical Security Plan.

In the same way, response should be included for routine matters in your other plans. However, there is a requirement for some specialized response plans. This should be limited to extremely dangerous incidents. Consider preparing such plans as a Bomb Threat and Response Plan; Fire Plan; Evacuation Plan; Natural Disaster Plan; Civil Disturbance Plan; and a Hostage Plan.

A Security Education Plan is appropriate as a separate plan if the size of your institution warrants it or if considerable emphasis is to be placed on security education. Otherwise, security education is best considered within your other plans.

Naturally, you will not be able to write these plans simultaneously. Here lies the need to prioritize their preparation and to answer the second part of the question posed earlier. Priority for plan preparation should be given to the most prevalent quantitative threats and the most critical threats. For example, a guard force usage plan, which includes individual guard orders, is best prepared before a bomb threat and response plan. The latter is certainly critical and life-threatening, but far less likely to be necessary (unless you are in a highly unusual situation) than the myriad incidents that your guard force may be called upon to prevent, detect, or respond to. This does not negate the need for a bomb threat and response plan, but does place it in a lower priority for preparation.

Plans are fine, but how well will they withstand the test of reality? It is hoped that you will never apply many of your plans, especially those dealing with emergency response. In the absence of an actual event, periodic testing and inspections are necessary, with special emphasis on testing. Testing should eliminate many doubts when realistic scenarios are used to validate the adequacy of your plans or to detect areas that need revision or strengthening.

The Cycle

All the steps have now been climbed, and a continuing cycle of security management may begin. Without the efforts that have gone into research, analysis, and planning, you would be unable to begin this cycle. The importance of those efforts cannot be overemphasized. You have established the basis for the continuing review of your security efforts and the modification of its objectives and procedures as the need should arise.

The foundation that has been laid includes people, equipment, a budget, and plans for dealing with security responsibilities. Your main security management efforts will now be to ensure that your plans, orders, and requests are carried out in a timely and effective manner. Naturally, there will be minor problems for you to contend with, but there should be no big surprises. Your effort will have been well spent and will allow you to perform with confidence.

NOTES

1. Joint Commission on Accreditation of Hospitals, *Accreditation Manual for Hospitals*, 1983 edition (Chicago IL: JCAH, 1982).

2. Timothy J. Walsh and Richard J. Healy, *Protection of Assets Manual* (Santa Monica, Ca: the Merritt Co., 1974).

3. Gion Green and Raymond C. Farber, *Introduction to Security* (Los Angeles, Ca: Security World Publishing Co., 1978).

4. *Physical Security*, Field Manual 19-30 (Washington, D.C.: Headquarters, Department of the Army, 1979).

Chapter 13

Personal Distress Devices for Health Care Personnel

Robert W. Doms, Sr., M.Ed.

The following event occurred in a federal medical treatment facility.

A nurse alone on duty at 1 a.m. in the alcohol dependence treatment ward was grabbed around the neck from behind by a patient. The patient gripped the narcotic cabinet key necklace worn by the nurse. As the necklace tightened around her neck, she pressed the transmitter alert button. Two medical center police on exterior patrols received the emergency signal directly on their portable radios, and the switchboard operator monitoring the central receiver and location readout display also received the signal. Central police responded in less than one minute, and serious injury to the nurse was prevented.

This terse account is void of emotion, but reflects the results that were desired and anticipated by concerned security personnel. If patient care personnel are required to work in environments where there is the possibility of physical assault, some means must be provided whereby they can summon assistance when required.

Prior to selecting a duress system, the health care administration must perform an objective evaluation of the facility.

1. Where are the risk areas? Is the risk area limited to one ward, one floor, the complete facility, or does it extend to the surrounding parking areas and facility grounds?
2. Who requires a duress alarm? Is the requirement limited to direct patient care personnel, or does it extend to maintenance, janitorial, and general support personnel?
3. In the event of an emergency situation, who would be able to respond?

4. In the event of an emergency situation, where would the request for assistance be received?

5. When does the threat exist? Is it present 24 hours a day, seven days a week, or is it limited to certain hours when staffing levels are minimal or to certain days when scheduled activity may invite assaultive behavior?

6. Can or should the system be used to monitor other events, such as unauthorized intrusion, fire, or temperature deviation?

7. If a system is selected that requires personnel to wear or carry individual transmitters, would the transmitters be acceptable to the personnel concerned? Some systems employ transmitters that weigh more than a pound, and while they are excellent devices for male personnel who can wear them on their belts, there is no practical means for affixing them to the typical uniform worn by female personnel.

8. What costs are involved? What is the initial acquisition cost? What are the terms and conditions of the warranty? What will it cost to have the system installed? Is a service contract desirable or required? Are service manuals available, and can the equipment be supported by the institution's maintenance personnel?

Upon obtaining the answers to these questions, the administration will be in a position to select or design a cost-effective system tailored to meet the majority of its requirements.

TYPES OF SYSTEMS

Duress alarm systems vary widely in price and complexity. The following discussion will classify them into three categories in ascending order of complexity and capability.

The least costly, but most often overlooked, is the hardwired system, consisting of strategically placed panic buttons installed throughout the threat area and hardwired to a monitoring site. A person requesting assistance depresses the closest switch, and a visual and/or audible alarm is received at a central location. This system can be used effectively in selected low-threat areas. The principal advantages are its lack of complexity and its nominal cost. But the acquisition cost, while minimal, may not be a true indicator of the final figure. Installation, if wiring is to be concealed and is required by local codes to run in conduit, may prove too expensive to justify the limited benefits provided by this system. Because of its simplicity, it requires little or no personnel training. Personnel simply need to know the location of the alarm switches.

This system can usually be installed by a facility's maintenance staff. Once a monitor site has been determined, a display panel should be designed to provide visual identification of the specific location or zone requesting help. This should be augmented with some form of audible identification that cannot be easily bypassed by monitoring personnel.

Most systems of this type operate on a low AC voltage. While most health care facilities have some type of emergency power system, power may not be available to the entire facility. Consideration should be given to a system designed to operate on DC power. Such a system could employ a rechargeable battery supply that constantly receives a trickle charge under normal conditions. When there is a power failure, the system would continue to function, powered by its battery supply. The drain rate is extremely low, so the capacity of the system does not have to be large or expensive.

A major disadvantage of the hardwired system is that the personnel must have access to one of the alarm switches, and if an individual were assaulted and unable to reach a switch, the system would be useless.

Another disadvantage is that because access to these switches is unrestricted, they can be activated by ambulatory patients who might mischievously initiate false alarms. This recently occurred in Memphis, where voluntary patients in a psychiatric holding area delighted in activating the alarms. The system is virtually free from falsing caused by mechanical malfunctions, but must be considered to have a potentially high false alarm rate due to maliciously initiated alarms. Regardless of the cause, falsing will rapidly defeat the effectiveness of any alarm system.

The next system is a satellite receiver system. Using a combination of radio frequency (RF) and hardwire, this system is more expensive, and offers more versatility. It consists of strategically located receivers mounted within the threat area. Each of the receivers is hardwired to a central monitoring console. Personnel are issued small duress alarm transmitters that are activated by squeezing. This sends a coded signal to a specific receiver. A receiver, when it detects the presence of its electronic identification code, closes a relay that activates the appropriate annunciator (lights, buzzer, or a combination) on the monitor panel.

The principal advantages of this system are its low acquisition cost and its flexibility. The transmitters are generally quite small, and personnel do not object to wearing them. If one is lost or damaged, its replacement cost is not excessive. The installation costs, again, may prove to be prohibitive, depending on local codes and construction techniques.

If the area to be monitored is not limited to a single ward, multiple receivers would be installed. To preclude interference and false alarms, each receiver would respond to one or more transmitters with ID codes that could be recognized by only one receiver. These low-power transmitters have a reliable range that is usually limited to 100 feet or less.

This system is less susceptible to malicious falsing and frees personnel from maintaining access to fixed alarm sites. The transmitters are in compliance with Part 15 of the Federal Communications Commission (FCC) *Rules and Regulations*. The user need not obtain a license or other form of approval from the FCC before purchasing or operating the system. Because of the limited number of frequencies that have been allocated for this use, the fact that no licensing is required, and the ready availability of these devices, it is likely that interference and falsing will increase as these systems become more widely used. The problem is similar to that experienced by users of Citizens Band (CB) radios. While this market is not expected to become as saturated as the CB market, the inability of the FCC to police and enforce its rules and regulations will increase if the current trend to reduce governmental regulation continues.

The last and most versatile system—the direct radio frequency—has the highest acquisition cost, but is the easiest and least expensive to install. It consists of a decoding receiver and a small standby power supply in one or more central monitoring sites. The system may be expanded to include a printer and a tape recorder that will record all emergency activity. A quantity of small alarm transmitters are worn by personnel who normally work in high risk areas. Several hundred of these transmitters can be used, and coverage usually extends throughout the entire facility and grounds. Most transmitters are lightweight and can be worn in leather belt-holsters or affixed to a nurse's uniform with a clip. One version now available weighs only seven ounces.

These transmitters are equipped with a shrouded panic button to prevent accidental activation. In the event of an emergency, the wearer depresses the panic button momentarily. This turns on the transmitter and sends a radio signal to the central monitor site, where a number identifying the specific transmitter in use is automatically displayed. An alarm is sounded to alert attending personnel, and a relay automatically starts a tape recorder that records all activity in the vicinity of the alarm transmitter. Each transmitter is equipped with an internal microphone. This audio capability offers two advantages: (1) the wearer can issue instructions and identify the specific type of assistance required, and (2) the exact location can be given.

Personnel responding to an alarm sounded by one of the systems discussed earlier have no way of knowing the nature of the emergency until they arrive on the scene. In the incident described at the introduction of this chapter, the duress transmitter worn by the nurse was on the same frequency as that used by the hospital security police. They monitored the emergency transmission, and, although they could not identify the ID number assigned to the transmitter, they were able to ascertain the location of the emergency and responded immediately without having to rely on dispatch information from the central monitor. The recording of this audio activity may become invaluable to the facility in the event of subsequent legal proceedings. These transmitters may also be equipped with a "deadman" switch. If the person wearing the transmitter is assaulted and knocked down, the transmitter will be activated automatically.

Although direct radio frequency systems are normally used in larger facilities or institutions with a substantial population of high risk patients, they can be considered as an effective multipurpose system for any facility, regardless of its size. They easily can be expanded to monitor other functions—a capability that should not be overlooked. Selective alarm transmitters, each with its own location identifying code, can easily be installed by security personnel to apprehend persons engaged in pilferage, trespass, and vandalism. Many different types of alarm transmitters are available for this purpose. Some have internal sensors, and others can be activated with any conventional N.O. (normally open) or N.C. (normally closed) sensor. All of these transmitters and the duress alarms can be monitored at one central location. Security and nursing staff are no longer required to monitor areas in person. The use of hardware in these instances in lieu of staffing is a very cost-effective technique.

As a health care provider or administrator, you must first identify the threat to your facility and its personnel to determine the level of protection that is needed. Then you can carefully design a system that will meet all of your objectives.

Administrators should not plan their systems based on the published sales data provided by vendors. An extensive onsite test of any proposed system should be conducted to determine the limits of reliable coverage. When performing these tests, it is important to duplicate actual operating conditions as closely as possible. Remember that all transmitters will not always be equipped with factory fresh, fully charged batteries. If you select a satellite receiver system, demand an extensive onsite test.

Next, review your results and amend your plan if necessary. It is also important to educate yourself and your coworkers concerning the purpose and operation of a duress system. The best personal distress devices will not provide protection if they are not used.

Chapter 14

Teaching the Management of Violent Behavior to Nursing Staff: A Health Care Model

John F. Moran, Ph.D.

The new nurse has just graduated. Whether leading to a bachelor of science in nursing, an associate of arts, or a nursing diploma, a rigorous course of study has prepared the new nurse to begin delivering health care services directly to patients. The technical skills called for in approved curricula have been mastered. The new nurse is ready to begin the practice of nursing.

An examination of the curricula being used throughout the United States and other countries reveals that considerable attention has been given to developing professionals well prepared to provide quality nursing services. In all, nursing education presents a well-formulated model of student preparation.

AN INSTRUCTIONAL GAP

A major deficiency in the design of nursing curricula must be acknowledged. With all of nursing's commitment to human service and healing, there is a failure in the field to account for human error and humankind's more negative side. Nursing education acknowledges psychiatric problems, but fails to discuss some of the behavioral implications of those problems. In short, nursing education fails to train the nursing student to manage human hostility. Worse, little or no recognition is given to the development of consistent training packages that prepare students to defuse potentially violent confrontations. Where training does occur in this regard at all, it typically involves physical management of assaultive behavior and techniques for getting patients into restraints.

While nursing education has yet to make de-escalation procedures part of its curricula, professional nursing literature has shown a growing awareness that practicing nurses are not prepared to avoid or respond to people who are on the verge of becoming violent or assaultive. A review of the literature indicates a major need for programs that directly address the specific steps that can be taken to survive a hostile encounter. In Australia, the United States, Ireland, and the United Kingdom, nursing's leaders have called for this gap to be closed.

In April 1983, I presented the first seminar on violence and aggression management in Ireland and the United Kingdom. Representatives of the nursing and medical press of those countries urged the presenters and all nursing educators to take up the challenge of this unaddressed problem. The president of the Irish Board of Nursing, while addressing the Dublin session of the Aggression Management Program, decried the growing rate of violent acts directed against Irish nursing personnel. In London, at a nationwide seminar centering on the same issues of aggression management, representatives of the Royal College of Nursing expressed their frustration at the lack of preparation and continuing training given United Kingdom nurses and other health care institution personnel. Australian hospital security personnel have expressed a deep concern that their nurses simply are not prepared to respond to the threat of violence in their hospitals. Internationally, the pattern is reported to be the same. Where training has been given, it involves techniques of placing a patient in restraints or simplistic forms of hand-to-hand self-defense. Little or no attention has been paid to developing a basic package of skills that can be taught quickly to prepare nurses to confront angry, hostile, or potentially violent people. The use of self-control and other basic techniques for talking aggressors down have not been communicated to the nurse.

The task facing nursing educators is clear. But, identifying the problem is only the first step. The strategy must be to develop a system of response that is both learnable and effective when used by the typical nurse. Additionally, the solution must ensure that the average nurse will remember the basic techniques under circumstances that are not generally conducive to instant recall. The training must address the skills needed by the nurse to defuse a potentially violent confrontation before the physical act has occurred. If energy is spent on the design of a system of physical response to the violent act, then a message is given to the nurse that the emphasis is on reacting to the problem, rather than on preventing it. To change this message, the pages that follow teach the essential skills to prevent and de-escalate the hostile moment.

Throughout the earlier chapters of this book, you have been exposed to the types of violence that might be encountered in a health care setting. Detailed information has been given regarding the legal aspects of response and the liability issues attendant to failing to appropriately respond. The personality and mind-set of the patient has been examined. An attempt has been made to point out the risky posture that a health care institution assumes when it fails to acknowledge that violent behavior can occur and fails to take reasonable steps to assure that its personnel are prepared to respond to it.

What follows is a model of prevention and de-escalation, the utility of which lies in the determination that it works and is easily learned by nursing personnel. The validity of this model has been established by the reports of those who have used it successfully to lessen the frequency and impact of violent confrontations at their hospitals. The value of this model rests in its foundation on common sense and lack of sensational claims for 100 percent success.

A unique feature of the program is that its techniques, while designed for nursing personnel, can be used by all health care staff members who might encounter hostile behavior. The physician in the emergency room is just as vulnerable to attack as the best-trained nurse. The social worker or psychologist is subject to the same risks of violence as the nurse or physician. I strongly recommend that these training programs be made available to the entire health care team.

RESPONSE AND RESPONSIBILITY

R and R is a military abbreviation for rest and relaxation. For the trainer who needs to prepare nursing personnel to de-escalate potential violence, these letters are the mnemonic key to an entire response strategy. The core of this system, indeed the key component of successfully confronting and handling aggressive people, is having a response and internalizing responsibility for the outcome of the situation.

Response comes first in the strategy of confrontation management, because reality has taught that when potential or actual physical violence occurs, some response has to be made and someone has to make it. Interestingly, there are times when the decision to do nothing is the best response.

Responsibility is the second major component, because in each instance, someone must always be identified to be responsible. Too often, the identification and assignment of responsibility has been to the wrong participant in the aggressive incident. In the majority of reviewable cases, the occurrence or incident reports have clearly pointed out that the patients, visitors, or other nonstaff aggressors were at fault. These reports often contain such phrases as, "There was nothing I could do; the patient suddenly . . ."; "He just went nuts on me"; "It was a surprise attack. It all happened so fast." Response and responsibility are central in aggression management; at issue is the question of who must respond and who is responsible.

The answer is not generally popular. First, it points out that the responsibility for the outcome lies primarily with the individual nurse or staff person who confronts the hostile and aggressive person. Second, responsibility can rest with other staff present or available to assist in the de-escalation. Third, the institution in which the confrontation occurs is responsible for training its personnel how to deal with this type of situation. Finally, and only to the least extent, responsibility for the physical act itself rests with the aggressor.

The response must be initiated by the staff person charged with maintaining order and calming the hostile or violent person. Contrary to many of our past health care practices, during a confrontation between a health care worker and a hostile and potentially violent person, the health care worker who is in most immediate danger of attack, regardless of rank, is the person to choose to respond or not respond. Title or job description is secondary during a moment of potential aggression. Until the nurse, aide, or technician confronting the dangerous person decides that the immediate danger is past, the staff person must be allowed to direct the interaction without unrequested interference by superiors or higher-ranking health care professionals. The rationale for this prohibition of interference is that the individual confronting the subject is the person most likely to suffer injury first, cause injury to the aggressive patient or visitor, or make some mistake that might cause both of the above.

When prime responsibility rests with the professional staff, its role in the long run is more easily understood and defined. The nurse confronting the aggression-prone patient is primarily responsible for the outcome of the confrontation. This role of the confronting professional defines the task of the mediator.

The nurse, as mediator, does not make deals, vacillate, or misrepresent the hospital or the basic tenets of good nursing care. In this context, given the stresses, actions, postures, and language of the moment, the nurse will elicit, shape, accelerate, decelerate, cause, allow, influence, heighten, or relax the agitation of the person being confronted. The progression of the agitated person from verbally hostile to verbally aggressive to physically violent is mediated by the actions and efforts of the confronting nurse or other health care professional.

It is very important that during the first stages of any aggression management training program the trainees understand and accept the concept of the mediator. It is as mediator that they will choose the response that fits the circumstances of any given confrontation. The role of mediator allows the nurse to enter and proceed through the confrontation without having to base decisions on whether there will be a winner or a loser. By selecting the role of mediator as the basis for processing an aggressive situation, the nurse does not involve personal ego. The task is to work a situation through and not to seek some form of resolution that merely complies with organizational policy. The issues facing the mediator are too dangerous to to be viewed in such a limited manner. An individual who mediates—who draws to a positive conclusion—must consider the reports that refer to the multitude of mistakes that lead to aggression escalation.

What the nurse does or fails to do in the first few seconds sets the stage for the severity of the behaviors that will follow over the next minutes of the confrontation. During training programs, the question is asked frequently, why the stress on personal responsibility? The answer is that when a human being knows that blame or responsibility can be projected on someone else, an unconscious excuse for eventual failure may already be in place. The existence of an excuse for failure is a major psychological chink in the nurse's aggression management armor. It may allow the nurse to believe that failure to de-escalate or control can be explained away. The potential rationalization of responsibility does not mean that the nurse wants to cause injury or be injured. It does, however, seem to increase the probability that someone will be hurt.

REDUCING THE ODDS

Nurses and all health care staff members are told during training in aggression de-escalation techniques that the salaries of health care staff members will never be high enough to make injury on the job an acceptable condition of employment. The point of engaging in this type of training is to avoid injury to the nurse and to the aggressive patient or visitor. The better the nurse is prepared to manage hostility, the better are the odds that no one will be hurt. A good preparation in aggression management techniques acknowledges that one component of success in this arena is an awareness of the predictability of the consequences of certain acts. There is a great deal to be said for being sensitive to playing the odds as decisions are considered.

The successful response to potential violence or the process of de-escalating the violent moment can be viewed as an interaction between two or more persons and a series of probabilities. How can the mediator increase the odds of a satisfactory outcome to an aggressive incident? Students are presented with a simple circle divided vertically into two equal hemispheres (Figure 14-1). Students are asked to accept that all possible causes of aggression and hostility escalation are contained in the circle. The left hemisphere represents those behaviors and causes that are directly attributable to the aggressor. The right hemisphere represents those directly attributable to the mediator.

Trainees are told that the objective of aggression de-escalation training is to chip away at the perimeter of the circle. It is hoped that this will reduce the

Figure 14-1 Causal Agents in Agression

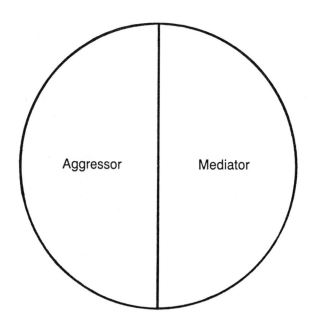

number of potential errors or causal agents that are exhibited during any given aggression confrontation. Unfortunately, it must also be pointed out that the behavior of the aggressor can only be controlled in an extremely limited number of ways. The aggressor may be physically restrained, chemically sedated, threatened into compliance, or in some way rendered unconscious. Short of these generally unacceptable alternatives, the nurse must rely on reducing personal error and thereby mediating a positive outcome of the confrontation. The circle can only be reduced by concentrating on the mediator's hemisphere. A chip is taken out of that side each time the mediator becomes aware of, and elects not to commit, an error during the confrontation.

In a formal training course, constant reference to this chipping away is recommended. If error is eliminated, the probability that physical violence will occur is proportionately reduced. This philosophy is expressed in Moran's Law: The greater the number of mediation errors made, the higher the probability of physical violence, and in Moran's First Corollary: Simple mistakes cause complex problems.

Simplicity

The nurse trained to de-escalate the aggressive moment will recognize the requirement to reduce the probability that violence will occur in each confrontation. While all behavior is caused, the individual staff person might not be aware of earlier actions or events that have predisposed the person being confronted to violence. No system and no form of training, however, can ever guarantee that its techniques correctly applied will reduce the probability of violence to zero. The mediator is responsible for reducing the odds to as close to zero as possible, without doing anything or allowing anything to happen that would increase the odds that the violent physical act will occur.

With a mandate to reduce the odds and to avoid simple mistakes, training then concentrates on the specifics of confrontation. What must the mediator do or not do when actually confronting the hostile or violent person? It is fortunate that most of what needs to be taught, people already know instinctively. This knowledge needs to be presented back to them in such a way that during a confrontation these actions are at a conscious level. During an aggressive incident, the nurse's immediate response must be the correct one. Without the time to plan, the staff person's response must be as good as if it had been planned. What develops then is a simple conscious response system that becomes immediately available for implementation.

Stance Is the Starting Point

During the late 1970s, management surveys were conducted within a major state's department of mental health facilities to determine where and how staff injuries occurred during violent confrontations. An interesting fact emerged. In the majority of reported cases, injuries did not occur just because staff were standing and confronting violent patients. The majority of injuries from assaults occurred once the staff nurse or psychiatric aide was no longer standing. Once the nurse had been knocked down, the seriousness of reported assaults increased. It appears that a victim who has been knocked down communicates a greater degree of vulnerability to an attacker, encouraging further violence. It also became apparent that no staff training had been reported that prepared nurses to confront violence-prone patients. Interviews with the victims of these attacks revealed the critical pieces of information. It was rare that the patient had pursued or had to make any great effort to hit the staff.

This survey pointed out what has remained a major training objective: to teach the nurse not only how to stand and remain standing when confronting the aggressor, but also what position to take to ensure that any blow does the least amount of damage. To accomplish this, the nurse stands with feet slightly spread, even with an imaginary line that might be drawn downward from the outside edge of the shoulders. This position, face to face with the aggressor, is called the basic balance stance. If the situation seems to become more tense, the nurse, without being too obvious, should move the dominant leg, usually the right, slightly to the rear with the knee unbent. The other leg should be slightly forward of the nurse's trunk and bent just a little at the knee. This position, the forward leaning stance, is extremely stable. The stability gained by going into this position will greatly reduce the odds of the nurse being knocked down by an initial blow.

During a training session, the students can pair off and face each other. One person plays the staff person and another the aggressor. The staff person first places both hands at the side and both feet close together. The person playing the aggressor places both hands on the staff person's shoulders and gently pushes backwards until the staff person loses balance. The roles are then reversed. The purpose of this simple exercise is to remind the trainees graphically how easy it is to lose balance with even slight pressure when one stands improperly. Trainees are instructed to assume a basic balance stance and then a forward leaning stance. The few minutes that staff spends in this activity help to eliminate the most common cause of severe staff injury.

With the ability to remain standing reinforced, the nurse is shown where to stand vis-a-vis the hostile person. Training conducted in the United States, England, and Ireland has confirmed that at least within these three nations the concept of body space and distancing remains constant. The nurse is shown how far to stand from the aggressor and where to stand relative to the aggressor's center and dominant side.

Mental health studies have shown that a significant number of injuries were related to blows to the nurse. The observation follows that

1. the blows did connect;
2. they connected solidly, doing damage; therefore,
3. the nurse was standing too close to the attacker.

Since all behavior is caused, it is important to examine what kinds of mistakes might have been made by the nurse that can be avoided by other nurses in similar situations.

Several conclusions can be drawn:

1. The nurse was within range of the attacker's blow; therefore, the distance between attacker and victim was approximately the attacker's arm length.
2. The nurse might have been close enough to the attacker to be within a discomfort zone that exists around all people.
3. The nurse may have given some aggression-provoking message to the aggressor that was or was not intended.

The question of intentional and potentially dangerous verbal language messages will be dealt with later. However, nurses being trained in de-escalation techniques frequently ask about these unintended messages. Since few people desire to be injured in an aggressive confrontation, it is safe to assume that most improper messages are given by accident, rather than by conscious decision. For example, aggressors might perceive nurses who stand too close and violate the comfort zone to be overconfident, challenging, or attempting to dominate. The nurse who stands too close may seem a threat to the angry person. During a confrontation with an angry and potentially violent person, one of the objectives is to avoid introducing any behavioral variables that cannot be reasonably predicted to assist in the de-escalation process.

The three earlier conclusions can be avoided if the nurse stands an arm's length and several inches from the aggressor. The arm's length must be that of the aggressor. This may place some burden on the nurse to become an accurate judge of such distances. At an arm's length plus several inches, the nurse tends to be outside the aggressor's discomfort zone, but still close enough to avoid making the impression that the nurse is frightened or unconcerned.

The nurse, while estimating the arm's length of the aggressor, must also make an immediate judgment about whether the aggressor is right- or left-handed. Once this determination is made, the nurse stands slightly off the aggressor's center and to the weaker or nondominant side. The basis for this placement is that a blow is most likely to come from the attacker's dominant hand or foot. By moving slightly off to the aggressor's weaker side, the nurse has maintained the appropriate distance from the attacker, kept a frontal pose, and increased the distance from the attacker's strong side. A blow that is struck toward this new position still may land, but the nurse is more likely to be hit during the follow-through of the strike.

An instant assessment of arm's length and handedness is not instinctual. There are ways, however, to increase the odds of a correct assessment of handedness. The nurse must remember these principles:

1. Nine out of ten people are right-handed.
2. A right-handed person is usually right-footed.
3. Most people will strike with their strong hand and kick with the foot on the same side.
4. Nine out of ten people wear wristwatches on their weak arms.
5. There is a greater than fifty-fifty chance that the tip of a person's belt points to the weak hand.

The nurse may also identify other accurate clues which may be added to the list above.

Why bother with standing in a certain way? Why worry about handedness? The answer goes back to Moran's First Corollary: Simple mistakes cause complex problems. It also brings up Moran's Second Corollary: The more times a potentially violent person is given the opportunity to attack, the more likely an attack will occur.

Stance and balance are only two components of the art of standing in confrontation with a hostile person. Role play exercises should instruct trainees regarding the use and placement of hands during an aggressive encounter. The two most important issues to be addressed are the tendency of nursing personnel to fold their arms over the chest and finger pointing and shaking.

Several elements are important to consider with regard to folding arms over the chest. First, most people cross the arms at the forearm and tuck one hand in front of and one behind the upper arm. This "double tuck" handicaps the nurse when a blow is struck and the nurse attempts to uncross the arms and move them into a more defensive posture. Second, when confronting a hostile person, folded arms should be avoided as it may convey a hostile, domineering, authoritative, or defensive body language message.

As a substitute, nurses should keep their hands at their sides and unclenched. There is a trick that is sometimes taught to public speakers that allows them to be comfortable with their hands at their sides. The technique is to have them tap the thumb with the forefinger of the right hand and then tap the thumb with the forefinger of the left hand. After several seconds, most people are totally unaware of their hands and are concentrating on other issues.

Many persons in health care have developed the unfortunate habit of using the index finger as a gestural method of emphasizing what they are saying. Unfortunately, this gesture is very frequently a contributor to hostility escalation. In no case in which the nurse is confronting the angry patient or visitor should finger pointing take place. In a program in which all efforts are made to reduce causes of aggression, such an obvious antagonistic gesture must be eliminated. The mediator who slips back into this habit will have expanded the circle of causal agents in aggression.

Eye contact is another form of body language that, if understood and used properly, can chip away at the circle of causes. It is often thought that the mediator must attempt to maintain as much eye contact as possible with the potentially violent person. The error of this belief rests in the inability of the nurse to predict the hostile person's response to this action. Constant eye contact can be very threatening under even the calmest of circumstances. There is no way to predict if the person being confronted interprets resolute eye contact as a challenging gesture. If aggressors have much sports experience, the possibility exists that they may use eye contact to fake a movement and draw the attention of the mediator from the real source of the movement or danger.

The situation may be further complicated if there is a marked difference in size between the nurse and the hostile person. If the mediator is taller than the aggressor, intense eye contact by the mediator may be interpreted by the aggressor as an attempt at dominance. If the mediator is shorter than the aggressor, then prolonged direct eye contact may be perceived as a sign of overconfidence or challenge. Trainees are reminded that these examples demonstrate that the mediator has the opportunity to remove potential sources of hostility escalation before they cause problems.

It is easy to recommend that people stop doing something. It is important that they have an alternate behavior in which they can engage. Common sense and some martial arts basics give the mediator an alternative target for eye contact. While glancing from time to time at the aggressor's eyes, attention needs to be directed primarily to an imaginary spot on the upper chest approximately where the first button down from the collar would be. Attending to this spot keeps mediators aware of any attempt at movement while also allowing their peripheral vision an opportunity to monitor the aggressor's hand movements. If movement is attempted, it will be observed, allowing some margin of readiness.

Control of Self Precedes Control of the Situation

The greatest resource in aggression confrontation situations is the mediator's mind. During attempts to reduce the probability of aggression escalation, the greatest amount of error is reduced by the nurse remaining outwardly and truly calm. The mediator accomplishes this by deciding to be calm. Unconsciously, the mind takes over, controlling various physiological systems to cause this mental decision to become a physiological fact. Under even the most stressful situations, the human mind has a remarkable capacity to control even the most automatic body functions. The mediator needs to be trained in techniques that assure control over muscle tension and respiratory rate and depth. In essence, the mediator is establishing and using a very positive "Pygmalion effect" to make the expectation of calmness ensure real calmness.

Muscle Tension

When a confrontation is anticipated or in progress, it is normal to tense various muscle systems. When this occurs, sometimes the aggressor is more aware of the mediator's tension than is the mediator. This may convey a message to the aggressor that the mediator cannot afford to transmit. It may say, for example, that the staff person is expecting an attack. When this type of message is received by a person already disposed by anger toward violence, the negative "Pygmalion effect" can occur. That is, when one expects something bad to happen, it can be brought about by the expectation.

Physiologically, muscles tense when opposing sets of muscles are equally tightened. Nurses generally need not be reminded that an arm movement, for example, takes place when one muscle is relaxed while the opposing muscle contracts. In a state of tension, both sides of a muscle group are tightened. Not only might the aggressor be given the wrong message, but at a moment when the mediator most desperately needs to be able to move quickly, micro-seconds are lost when one side of a muscle group must be relaxed before the other can bring a limb into motion. If the nurse or staff person were tense and would need to move fast to a defensive posture, muscles would be fighting each other to come out of the tensed state. This additional micro-second delay of response could make the difference between injury or evasion of injury.

To prepare mediators to assess their tension levels, a simple exercise is recommended. Self-monitoring can be done under two very different sets of circumstances. First, on the next occasion when the trainee becomes angry or tensed, time should be taken to attempt to bring to a conscious level the feelings that are being experienced. If a mirror is available, the nurse could go to it and see what signs of muscle tension would be obvious to a person being confronted. If this is difficult to do, students are advised to look at their own faces in a mirror during a stress-free moment of privacy. The facial muscles that are tightened in times of tension or anger are usually revealed by permanent wrinkles that appear around the eyes, nose, and mouth. The mediator must practice relaxing these facial muscles on mental command. As another exercise, the mediator might try to make an extremely tight fist with the dominant hand and hold that fist to the verge of discomfort, then slowly open the hand. The softening feeling then experienced is that of a muscle relaxing. The mediator should seek a similar feeling in all the major muscle groups when tension is perceived during an aggression confrontation.

Controlled Breathing

Attempting to remember everything that needs to be done during an aggression confrontation requires clear and quick thinking, which in turn requires a constant flow of oxygen to the brain. If the mediator's respiratory rate increases and the depth of respiration becomes more shallow, not only is the supply of oxygen to the brain reduced, but the pitch and volume of the voice goes up. All of these consequences of stress increase the probability of error.

An example of this occurred within a large hospital in which a security officer was "written up" by three different administrators for a surly attitude toward hospital staff members confronted during the course of a vehicular patrol. The director of security, knowing that this was a good officer and a person who generally interacted well with other employees, rode as an observer on the next patrol. The director observed that each time the officer exited the vehicle to confront a staff person who had violated a traffic regulation, the officer would immediately become tense. Exiting the vehicle and walking to the other car, the officer would begin breathing more rapidly and shallowly. It was obvious that this type of confrontation was very difficult for the officer, who disliked the role of enforcer and preferred protecting and serving fellow employees. During these tense moments, the officer's voice would become loud, shrill, and very high-pitched, like the sound of fingernails on a blackboard. The quality of the officer's voice incited hostility. The content of this officer's verbalizations was almost irrelevant. The cure was quick and simple. The officer was trained to monitor breathing while approaching employees. In this way, the officer learned to retain control and remain calm. In the end, both the officer and the staff members to be corrected interacted calmly and rationally.

It is important for staff members who are going to act as mediators in aggression de-escalation to learn the techniques used by that officer. The essence of the technique is that the mind controls the body. Trainees are taught to literally talk to themselves as they approach and confront. On approaching the angry patient or visitor, nurses must ask themselves, "Am I breathing too rapidly? Am I breathing too shallowly?" They must answer internally and immediately. If the answer is yes, then the nurses must consciously slow their breathing, increase depth of their respiration, and give themselves a reminder that the situation is under control and that they must be calm. Mediators thus talk themselves into calmness and control. This self-questioning and answering is absolutely essential. When it is carried out, the staff person will become calm. When mediators can think clearly and quickly, there will be less doubt whether their stances are correct, whether their distances from aggressors are adequate, and whether they are talking in low and calm voices.

If the mediator doesn't carry out this internal conversation, some of the de-escalation procedures may be forgotten. Forgetting could lead to failure. The price of failure here is that someone will get hurt.

As a director of security, I once was summoned to confront a psychiatric patient armed with a knife and threatening to kill any staff member that came near. Approaching this person and using these procedures, it occurred to me how silly it would look if the trainer managed to get himself killed using his own techniques. The first idea I had was to play ten-cent psychologist and ask the patient if he was mad at me. Because I was monitoring myself, I had the presence of mind to tell myself how stupid that particular question would be. The patient was obviously already angry, and since I was the only person present, I instantly would have drawn the focus of all of his anger toward myself. Instead, I asked the patient's name and gave my own in return. Instead of drawing anger, I put us on the level of two people with first names.

The point of this story is that this self-questioning and answering can be accomplished in micro-seconds and can help the mediator avoid tragic errors. A benefit derived from the internal monitoring process is the heightened ability of the mediator to be aware of and assess the emotional state of the hostile person and the environment in which the confrontation is occurring.

As mediators approach hostile persons, they must maintain the posture and demeanor of individuals who are interested and who will try to help. Speaking and standing calmly, mediators should remain balanced and ready to move. The pitch and volume of their voices must be lowered. Speech should be clear and slow. Simple and precise words must be used that will be immediately clear to the listener. The language used must be polite, devoid of profanity or threat. At the same time, no childish derivatives of common expletives should be spoken. Using words such as heck or darn can imply a weakness on the part of the mediator. Simple, straightforward communication will work best.

Simultaneously, the mediator should look for early warning signals of emotional instability or impending attack. Signs of excessive adrenalin production and muscle tension must be noted. Are the aggressor's fingers, eyelids, or other muscles twitching? Does the person being confronted withdraw at all as the mediator approaches? Is there any change in the posture of the hostile person? Is the confronted person looking around the room for an exit, a corner, or a weapon? Does the aggressor seem to reduce the distance between the participants? All of these observations provide critical information to the mediator. An appreciation of this data is important in reducing the number of things that can go wrong during the confrontation. The ability to make these observations, process them for their relevance, and act accordingly, all in a matter of seconds, depends on clear thinking. This form of thought will be possible in such stressful encounters only when the mediator's mind is in control of all basic bodily systems.

The benefits of clear thinking extend into the moments of a confrontation in progress. Trained staff members are aware of the extreme danger in cornering a hostile or violent person. More important, clear-thinking staff members are sensitive to and avoid all four types of cornering. Too often, people only think of the most common type, angular cornering.

Staff members need to be alert to three other types of cornering as well:

1. Angular cornering is the placement of the individual in the angle formed by two walls or objects. The hostile person is trapped. The only way out for the aggressor is over the body of the mediator.
2. Exit cornering is a form of cornering in which the hostile person cannot escape the presence of the mediator without first approaching the mediator and reducing the distance between the two parties. This form of cornering puts a price on disengagement. The nurse may give the impression to the aggressor that "it's permissible to disengage, but to do so you have to reenter my (the nurse's) sphere of control one more time before you can leave." When having successfully calmed a hostile person, the mediator blocks the exit or stands too close to it, this is exit cornering at its worst. This greatly increases the odds of renewed agitation and violates Moran's Second Corollary when it gives the aggressor an additional and unnecessary opportunity to attack. Staff members need to remember that if aggressors have to reduce the distance between themselves and the authority figure in order to leave that person's presence, then exit cornering is taking place. When the new minimum distance is reached between the aggressor and mediator, the moment of greatest likelihood of renewed hostility has been reached.
3. Psychological/verbal cornering is based upon the premise that human beings, even when emotionally distraught, tend to respond to opportunities to disengage when it appears to be in their best interest to do so and when it is possible with minimal loss of face. Mediators can minimize loss of face for aggressors by giving them the impression that they are free to choose from among at least two courses of action. Experience with psychiatric and developmentally disabled patients and normal juveniles and adults has shown that when given options

for subsequent behavioral choices, individuals choose those that are most socially and personally safe. When people are ordered to do something, however, there is a strong tendency, even in the calm person, to make the more rebellious choices.

Nurses have to learn to be cautious about making commands. If the mediator tells the hostile person to "stop that and sit down," any or all of the following could occur:

a.   If an audience is present, there is little likelihood that the aggressor will obey.

b.   Even without an audience, the nurse has set up a situation where the odds are fifty-fifty that the aggressor will simply refuse.

c.   A command too often is challenging and implies that there will be a winner and a loser.

No matter what the reason for the hostile person's noncompliance, the aggressor did not set up this component of the confrontation. The mediator did. If the aggressor says no to an order, the options for the mediator's next move are fairly limited. Does the mediator then force compliance or back down? In neither case is there a winner.

4.   Contact cornering occurs when the mediator grabs or holds the hostile person. In order to grab someone, the nurse must obviously get very close to the target. The issue of distancing surfaces again. The mediator was cautioned earlier about appropriate distances. In the act of grabbing and holding a person, all safeguards and sensitivities to body space are ignored. Once the mediator has grabbed the aggressor, an extremely strong body language message is given. The intensity of the grasp is not the only factor involved. The aggressor, by virtue of being grabbed, has only two choices: submit to the will of the person grabbing or resist. Once an angry patient or visitor has been grabbed by the mediator, the probability of physical aggression is fifty-fifty or worse. The accompanying risk of physical injury to one of the participants is increased by the proximity and the intensifying effect of the physical transmission of intent.

The danger of physical contact—grasping, grabbing, holding—does not eliminate those activities from the behavioral repertoire of the mediator. It does, however, suggest that it be used only when absolutely necessary and only as a planned response to the demands of the situation. Certain techniques can reduce some of the danger. The nurse can explain to the patient or visitor exactly what is about to occur. The nurse might say, "I am going to take your arm. I need to do this because . . . ."

Sometimes, the best way to handle a disruptive situation is to combine several of the techniques reviewed here. At one Illinois hospital, the unit director for the psychiatric floor shared techniques that his nursing personnel used with patients who refused required and prescribed medications. A refusal to take medications creates a difficult situation for the nursing staff. The physician has ordered the medication for the patient's best interest. The nurse is required to follow the physician's orders. The policy on that unit is that if the patient refuses to cooperate with the physician's orders, the unit director or shift supervisor will advise the patient that there are only so many minutes in which to choose to take the medication either orally or by injection. It is pointed out to the patient that the manner of administration is of no concern to the nurse. The staff simply has a job to do—to see that prescribed medications are administered. The patient is told that if the deadline is reached and the medication has not been taken orally, it will be assumed that the patient has knowingly decided in favor of an injection. Once the deadline has arrived, even if the patient faced with an injection voices a preference for oral administration, the medication is administered by injection. The injection is preceded by a matter-of-fact observation that the patient chose this route of administration by the behavior exhibited. Staff administering the injection do so with complete regard for patient comfort, but also with a firm determination to follow through on the option indicated by the patient's behavior. It is rare on this unit that this procedure is ever engaged in more than once with a given patient. It has also been equally rare on this unit that any physical aggression has followed this very well-planned interaction.

The technique of allowing the aggressive person to choose an act and, therefore, its consequence, is more helpful than one might realize. In formulating an order so that the aggressive person sees compliance as a choice, rather than as submission, the mediator has eliminated the elements of both of their egos.

Distraction, Cognitive Dissonance, and Incompatible Responses

Simple actions can sometimes work better than the most elaborate strategies. The mediator is reminded of the potential value of controlled distraction during the confrontation. The mediator might offer to provide the hostile person some privacy, a soft drink, or just a place to sit and talk. One hospital keeps bogus forms in the waiting room of the emergency department that the mediator and the frightened or hostile person can fill out together to distract the person from fear or anger by overwhelming the poor soul with bureaucratic paper work. The mediator rationalizes this distraction by explaining that these extensive history forms may offer some unexpected piece of medical or social history that could be of some use to the treatment team working with the visitor's family member (the patient). On successful de-escalation and dismissal of the patient or visitor, the forms are thrown away.

Whether by having a soft drink or by filling out bogus forms, the aggressive person is distracted from one or more of the sources of aggression stimulation. One cannot sit and consume a soft drink at a level of pre-violent readiness. Nor can one be working with a mediator filling out bogus forms and still be escalating at the same rate toward greater violence.

In much the same way, the staff person can use a technique called cognitive dissonance. Simply put, this means doing what the aggressor least expects the mediator to do. A member of my staff, a five-foot, five-inch eight-year veteran of Illinois' Cook County Hospital Emergency Room, prides in telling the story of the time when a six-foot, six-inch irate 300-pound male confronted her in a treatment cubicle and informed her that he was going to kill her right there while they were alone. This patient was between the nurse and the doorway. The nurse responded to this chilling threat with robust laughter as she looked back and forth between her small frame and the patient's bulk. Apparently, her perception of the humor in the hopelessness of the situation surprised the would-be attacker. The contrast in the sizes was all too apparent. The patient joined in the laughter and the nurse was able to talk her way out of the situation. What would have happened if the nurse had resisted, frozen in fear, or backed further into a corner? No one will ever know. Will laughter always work? It's doubtful. When asked why she chose this response, the nurse revealed that it was the only response that came to her mind at the time. It turned out to be the one response that the aggressor didn't expect.

On another occasion, I was present in the emergency room of a midwestern hospital when a distraught father carried in his six- or seven-year-old daughter who had obviously serious leg injury. The parent stood for some time at the ward clerk's desk, holding the crying child in his arms. The ward clerk never even looked up, but continued with the paper work on the desk. This seemed to go on for a long time. In a totally empty emergency room, this hospital employee kept the patient and father standing for no apparent valid reason. The father was becoming visibly more tense and angry by the second. It was only when the father became verbally threatening that nursing personnel were summoned to begin treatment of the child. The hostility of the father was not decreased by the removal of the child to an adjoining treatment area, because he could still hear her crying and assumed that the experience he had just gone through was in some way continuing out of his sight. A nursing supervisor walked in on this situation, did a two-second appraisal, and said, "Your daughter is with the best of some of my people;

how about I get us some coffee?" The break in tension and hostility was so strong it could almost be felt. This distraction, an unexpected act of kindness, instantly dispelled the aggression.

ALTERNATIVE ENDINGS

The examples just given, and others that nurses have lived through, could all have ended differently. They could have ended with nurses seriously injured. They could have ended with otherwise normal, non-violent persons acting out in such a way as to cause the destruction of hospital property or the injury of patients, visitors, or other participants. But they didn't, and 99 percent of aggressive encounters don't have to escalate beyond the point when the nurse enters as mediator.

The de-escalation of the violent encounter requires a response made by a nurse or other health care professional who recognizes the responsibility that goes with the profession. The response is based on previously considered strategies and an awareness of the dynamics of human confrontation.

The training recommended in this chapter represents a blend of clinical experience and an understanding of human behavior. Central to the success of this training model is the health care professional's awareness that people, no matter what their titles, will do under stress what they have been prepared to do. Without prior training, they do not know how to de-escalate human confrontation. Physicians, nurses, psychologists, social workers, or administrators who confront human aggression without proper preparation not only risk serious personal injury, but they risk liability of a different, but equally threatening, nature for the organizations they represent.

Chapter 15

Treatment of Staff Victims of Violence

Gail Pisarcik Lenehan, R.N., M.S., C.S., C.E.N.
and James T. Turner, Ph.D.

Only recently has reliable data on institutional violence begun to be evaluated seriously, and there is every indication that the problem is significant. Data from the National Institute of Justice shows that at least one-third of the individuals in large urban areas will be victims of violence. The percentage for women is even higher. As has been discussed throughout this volume, the risk of violence by patients, families, and outsiders has not bypassed health care systems. Even with increased security, attacks continue. At times, employees have signed petitions demanding tighter security, protested a lack of security, admitted to carrying revolvers to work, and declined to be hired, creating staffing problems.[1] As mentioned in Kenneth Tardiff's chapter on the psychiatric patient, assaults have occurred against 42 percent of the psychiatrists surveyed.[2] When assaults are brought to light, silent suspicion or a recriminating finger is often directed toward the victim.

Staff members tacitly deny the problem. Under-reporting of assaults on staff members in a state hospital has been documented.[3] At a Veterans Administration neuropsychiatric hospital, the respondents, who had an average of six years of psychiatric nursing experience, reported being assaulted an average of seven times prior to the study period.[4] Even the patients and lay public seem to take assaults for granted. This attitude is typified by one female patient's response in a study[5] of why patients use the emergency department: people who were sick sometimes had to show it and the emergency department had to stand for that kind of thing, because that's what they are there for. A male patient's remarks echoed this conclusion. He felt that emergency department staff "had to take a lot of———. That's what they're there for."[5]

In a study of a neuropsychiatric hospital by Lanza,[4] a large number of staff members indicated they had no reactions to an assault. Some indications existed that staff members felt they would be overwhelmed if they allowed themselves to admit their feelings. Because assault was an acknowledged risk in their positions, some felt they had no right to react. Interestingly, Sales, Overcast, and Merrikin[6] indicate that unless employees or contractors are specifically hired to deal with violent behavior, they have no reason to anticipate assault as a routine part of their employment. This attitude of minimizing the impact of assaults is not limited to health care staffs. In a study of patients referred to a special clinic for the treatment of stress response syndromes, only 10 percent ever came for treatment.[7] In this light, staff victims may not recognize the need for help or they may feel that seeking help would be just another blow to their self-esteem. We often admonish patients for neglecting physical and emotional conditions; the question arises whether we need to heed the admonition to heal thyself.

In this chapter's title, the word treatment is used for expediency. It may be the wrong word to use with respect to helping staff members. All victims suffer some loss of self-esteem, but for staff members in a helping institution, victimization in their own work settings may lead to especially deep narcissistic wounds. The term treatment may reinforce an image of lowered status. Treatment is given to one who is not self-sufficient; this is clearly at odds with many health care providers' self-images. Staff members are accustomed to helping, not being helped. Being patient-like is to be vulnerable, powerless, laughable, pitiable, ignorant, or noncompliant. Primarily, you are different. The useful emotional barrier that staff members erect between themselves and patients begins to crumble. This barrier, which protects staff members from overidentification and its consequent anxiety, is impaired when a staff person takes on the dual role of staff member and patient.

Victim is another term used with some reservation. This particular label is one with which few want to be burdened. In the case of a serious physical or sexual assault, the label of victim can create a terribly onerous new identity— a whole new person. "That's the one who got attacked," some whisper as they watch the individual's behavior more closely. One victim captured this new identity: "I feel like a freak. People watch me now—even my own family. They treat me differently. I don't know what they expect me to do."

REACTION OF VICTIMS

Lists of victims' symptoms have been compiled.[4,7] These usually include combinations of emotional, biophysiological, and interpersonal reactions. This chapter will address a few symptoms that are more directly linked to the recovery of staff members and the quality of patient care.

Labeling

The cognitive activity of labeling bridges all the factors in victims' responses. First, as discussed, labeling with the word victim begins an erosion of healthy self-image and self-esteem. Second, because those called victims are different, a distancing from significant others begins. Victims begin to see themselves and their reactions in a more negative light. They may begin to feel that they were attacked because they were different or that they are now different because they were attacked. Reinforcing this attitude are the unconscious needs of other staff members to fend off anxieties over their own vulnerability. "I am different from the victim, therefore it couldn't happen to me."

Distancing by Others

Victims may feel that others now relate to them differently. This may be true. Staff members who are assaulted may be seen as provocative or otherwise at fault. They may be selectively remembered as abrupt and angry with patients—asking for trouble. One of the authors observed a judge begin the questioning of a health care staff member who was pressing assault charges against a patient by asking, "What did you do to provoke the patient?" The case was dismissed. Such thoughts reinforce the very comforting "just world" theory—people get what they deserve and deserve what they get. Most people subscribe to this myth on some level, and medical care staff members are no exception. Blaming the victim—unconsciously or otherwise—distances others from that victimization. If that distance is suddenly removed, the stark awareness of one's vulnerability, even fragility, could be overwhelming. Interestingly, it appears that the more seriously hurt a staff member is, or the more compromising and embarrassing the assault, the more others will perpetuate the victimization. This separateness may occur by omission—by failing to mention the obvious or to acknowledge that any unusual event has occurred.

Emotional Disturbance

Major symptoms found in victimized staff members can be grouped into three areas: anger, fear, and depression.

Anger after an assault arises from several legitimate considerations. First, the violent patient may receive secondary gains from other staff members. For example, a patient in an emergency department was rapidly assessed as not appropriate for the hospital admission which she demanded. The patient then attacked the nurse who was discharging her. As a result of the assault, a consulting physician was called. This action had previously been denied to the patient. The physician and another nurse spent the next three hours evaluating the patient and finally admitted her. Violence had helped her reach her stated goal of hospitalization, while staff members undercut the assaulted nurse. In another situation, a general medicine patient was treated with new respect and deference by clinic personnel after she assaulted a staff member with whom she'd had a disagreement.

A second source of anger is the lack of adequate protection. Security measures may have been absent or inadequate. Other staff members may not have responded appropriately during the assault, or their actions may have placed the victim in danger. Physicians may have minimized nurses' and aides' evaluations of danger and refused to order restraints. All these issues contribute to the victim's anger. Therefore, consideration of these issues needs to be included in any assessment and treatment of staff victims.

Reactions of fear and anger in staff members can interfere with the effective management of the aggressive patient. Patients who act out angry feelings can elicit both fear and anger in health care personnel. Staff members are clearly capable of responding in their own way to fear, anger, and anxiety.[8] Staff members, for example, may insist on premature discharge or transfer. When staff members feel that direct expression of anger toward assailants is inappropriate, they may find indirect methods of expression. If methods of expression are not found, feelings of powerlessness and frustration will increase.

Depression is an alternative to outwardly directed anger. Staff members can depreciate their biophysiological symptoms of depression. Such clinical symptoms of depression after violent episodes are not uncommon and include the following:

- sadness
- poor appetite
- sleep disturbance
- lowered self-esteem
- decreased motivation
- fatigue
- crying spells
- irritability
- feelings of emptiness

The loss of one's safety is significant. Victims need to mourn the loss of their feelings of security and, by extension, their immortality and control.

Involving both fear and depression is the common occurrence of an obsession with the violence. In an attempt to restore control and order, the victim needs to review details of the assault for clues or causes. The "if onlys" need to be gone over repeatedly by victims of violence before they are forgotten.[9] The "if onlys" invariably point to self-blame. Victims try to assure their future safety by ascribing this blame. This attempt to use the past to control the future occurs because it is too burdensome to think an assault might happen anywhere or anytime, even at work. When this obsessing occurs, it is valuable to allow the victim freedom to review details and the "if onlys." Significant others may find it too tedious or too painful to listen to these repetitive themes.

Biophysiological reactions accompany these reactions. They may include the following:

- headaches
- body tension
- appetite/sleep disturbances
- increased startle responses

All of these reactions can lead to a decline in the quality of health care delivery. The physician who is too anxious to get close to patients may perform inadequate physical examinations. Nurses may fail to monitor vital signs accurately. Aides may overlook basic care needs of troublesome patients or patients who evoke memories of a past assault.

TREATMENT OF VICTIMS

Approaching Victims

Staff members will be acutely aware and sensitive to the manner in which help is offered. They will be attuned not only to the content of communications, but also to pity, condescension, or subtle implications that the assaults were provoked. Re-victimization can easily occur during this particularly impressionable time. Peer support on an informal basis is an ideal. Unqualified empathic support is highly important.

Immediate Intervention

As with many crises, early, informal intervention can set a tone for a better resolution. Victims of violence need help with immediate problem solving and decision making. This might involve determining the extent of injuries and the need for treatment; preparing formal medical-legal reports; providing immediate transportation; ensuring that the victim is not alone at home for a short period after the incident (if the situation warrants); and ensuring that one person from the health care facility assumes responsibility for keeping in touch with the victim during any absence. Whom to tell about the assault and the issue of pressing criminal charges may be content areas that the victim needs assistance in exploring.

Precautions

Attention to and concern for the victim's assault experience is occasionally a double-edged sword. The staff member who is already stressed may find in this attention and concern a reason to regress, withdraw, or act out other unresolved issues. Conveying an expectation of emotional debilitation may be a self-fulfilling prophecy. Support, as opposed to therapy, can set a tone for initial intervention that subtly implies an expectation of evolving mastery and strength without minimizing the situation.

Support Versus Professional Counseling

There is a line (albeit a thin one) between support and professional counseling. A helping person needs to be cognizant of when that line is crossed. An incident of violence is a very personal event, and personal issues are always involved. However, some staff victims may need or want to discuss the situation and their reactions within the context of work and professionalism and choose not to see the assault or hostage taking as a personal affront. This desire is best respected and validated both directly and indirectly. If the individual wishes to view the violence within the professional realm, support is the intervention of choice. The choice to distance the violence from oneself as a person may arise from the collective view of violence by the staff as a whole in a particular setting. The reaction to violence by a general medicine patient in full contact with reality may be radically different from the reaction to violence by an acutely psychotic psychiatric patient. Violence is expected and tolerated to different degrees depending on whether the setting is public or private, outpatient or inpatient, medical or psychiatric.

TREATMENT ISSUES

Support

Health care staff members who are victims of violence have the same difficulties in overcoming fear and phobic reactions as other victims. Staff members are burdened with heightened fear and suspicion. People who normally think very positively find themselves with immediate reactions of distrust, thinking that others will inflict harm if given the chance. They are hypervigilant. The intensity of this fear seems to abate with time. Victims need to be reassured that these characteristics of hypervigilance—the pounding heart and trembling body at the sight of someone who resembles the assailant or wears similar clothes—are normal following such an incident.

The anxieties may be free-floating, often accompanied by an increased startle response. A book drops, the victim jumps. Minor issues become sources of irritation. Nightmares involve re-creations of the violence. Dreams of helplessness increase. The need to seek refuge with trusted friends or family occurs with an emphasis on a sense of safety. Victims, even professionals, need to be reminded that these are normal responses to crises.

Anger is an important and complex treatment issue. Anger may be repressed, suppressed, or denied. Invariably, anger does surface. However, it may be displaced to people other than the assailant. Offers of support may serve as lightning rods for the initial bursts of anger. Beyond that, however, professional therapy is needed to reconstruct and restructure the anger. Psychodynamic therapy may be called for if the anger is linked to past experiences to intensify personal conflicts. Other types of psychotherapy may be necessary to help the victim integrate the experience and close the chapter.

Victims may often find themselves unable to control these intense emotions and push away from personal friends and co-workers who could provide support.

Significant others in the victim's social and work structures may need professional intervention as well so that they can maintain their supportive stance of the victim. Displaced anger can lead to verbal rejection: "How could you let me work in a hospital in such a bad neighborhood? You're never there when I need you. I don't want to stay anymore." Relationships with colleagues and co-workers can be severely disrupted. Significant others may need counseling and assistance to develop concrete plans on how to relate, how to handle emotional reactions, whether they be anger or crying spells, and how to handle feelings of awkwardness and avoidance.

Treatment

There is no consensus regarding the best treatment modality for health care staff members who are victims of violence. An appropriate goal in crisis intervention[10] is to return the victim to the premorbid base line. A basic assumption for this type of intervention is that the victim is essentially a normal individual. If there is evidence otherwise, in-depth psychotherapy is a more appropriate treatment. The Chinese symbol for crisis represents opportunity as well as danger. By coping with a personally traumatic situation successfully, one turns the crisis into an opportunity for growth and change. Emotional, biophysical, and interpersonal responses need to be addressed in treatment. Different psychotherapeutic techniques appear useful in crisis intervention with staff victims of violence. One of the difficulties has been organizing the treatment plan so that it covers the multiplicity of emotional, biophysical, and interpersonal symptoms. Sank[11] offers an interesting method for organizing the types of problems and types of treatment. He uses a multimodal profile[12] to isolate areas for change: behavior, affect, sensation, imagery, cognitions, interpersonal relations, and drugs. This method can be used to assess the victim's multiple symptoms and determine appropriate treatment.

For example, such cognitions as "I was assaulted, therefore, I am ineffective and powerless" could be confronted through cognitive/reality therapy. Human beings are constantly in search of meaning. The fantasized meaning of an assault may need to be explored, since this meaning may predicate, in part, the victim's response to the violence. Mental images may require a gestalt or reconditioning model. Each of the problem areas can lend itself to unique intervention techniques.

Whatever the modalities that are assessed and the techniques used, a basic groundwork in all treatment is a matter-of-fact acknowledgment of the violence. While others may have tried to ignore the incident or felt awkward broaching the subject, it is essential that the support source or the treatment professional remove some of the emotional charge from the subject of violence by directly asking about the physical and emotional impact.

Respecting Psychological Defenses

Helping persons should always remember that staff members who are victims of violence are not unlike victims of sexual assaults. They may not be seen as, or feel like, real victims with all the secondary gains that the victim role offers. Victims may be unable or unwilling to accept the identity of "victim," let alone seek help. In an attempt to flee their illegitimate status, many psychological defenses may be employed to minimize, erase, negate, or magically undo the event. "It wasn't that bad; I'm not really hurt; No big deal; I'm not going to cry over spilled milk; It could have been worse; I could be dead." The need to regain one's dignity and bring life back to normal is strong. These quickly mounted defenses are best dealt with gently by the helping individual. Interventions that weaken the defenses too quickly may cause more damage than good. In these crises, a major part of the victims' present and future armamentarium is the defenses and coping mechanisms they have developed over a lifetime. In contrast to traditional in-depth psychotherapy, extended attention to an act of violence and elicitation of affect may exacerbate the situation. The best barometer of whether to go further and explore deeper feelings when helping a victim is the effectiveness of the current defense structure. If the defenses employed are effective and allow the victim to productively cope, leave the structure alone. If, however, they are ineffective, counterproductive, and produce other problems, then attempts at change are clearly indicated.

ADMINISTRATIVE ISSUES

Time off from the job seems to be helpful for most victims. Removing the victim from the situation for a short time helps the healing of psychic as well as physical wounds. If sanction is not given, more prolonged absenteeism may result. "Time out," an alternative or supplement to time off, allows individuals to work in different areas or with different groups of patients until they feel comfortable returning to their primary work areas. It may be particularly difficult for victims to return to inpatient units where the violent patient may still be present.

For those in fields in which caring and giving are the order of the day, a certain positive regard for patients and people is important. That positive regard is significantly threatened by violence. Some staff members will never feel comfortable in the same situations. To try to overcome intense fears may be futile and counterproductive. Treatment will not improve symptomatology when wounds seem to be reopened in daily situations that engender fear. Objective guidance and exploration of career options may be best. Leaving a position is not necessarily an admission of weakness or defeat, but simply part of taking good care of oneself.

Staff-wide Interventions

Other staff members' interest and curiosity about the incident and their need to protect themselves are best addressed in an already existing forum, such as a staff meeting. A psychological "autopsy" of the event may allow a sharing of feelings and a discovery of options for increased assurance of safety. The leader can set a tone of empathy, comradery, and humor. Nonsensational, dignified, and humorous descriptions can help to reframe and relabel the experience so that it is more tolerable and more easily integrated for everyone. The victim, if willing, may be deferred to as an expert. Setting a tone for others' respectful responses can help increase low self-respect after victimization.

In some cases, treatment may be wise for a large number of staff members not themselves the direct victims of violence. Bursten et al.[13] arranged group meetings to assist such staff members after a hostage taking at a children's hospital. Significant numbers of nurses and nurses' aides reported increased anxiety, dreaming, fear, and other stress symptoms. A similar group treatment strategy was used by Sank[11] in addition to individual sessions. These interventions appeared useful and cost-effective.

CONCLUSION

The appropriate support and reinforcement of coping strategies for staff victims of violence is a very subtle and challenging business—a business we need to know much more about. It is interesting that little data in general exists about the outcome of violence in health care as it relates to staff members. What has happened to the large number of physicians mentioned in Kenneth Tardiff's chapter? Why does what little is available deal with nursing? Does the past sex stereotyping of professions—nurse (female) and physician (male)—have anything to do with the permissibility of after-violence reactions? If charity begins at home, these issues certainly deserve our attention.

NOTES

1. R. R. Rusting, "Introduction," *The Health Care Security Crisis Handbook* (Port Washington, N.Y.: Rusting Publications, 1984).

2. D. J. Madden, J. R. Lion, and M. W. Penna, "Assaults on Psychiatrists by Patients," *American Journal of Psychiatry* 133 (1976): 422-425.

3. J. R. Lion, W. Snyder, and G. L. Merrill, "Underreporting of Assaults on Staff in a State Hospital," *Hospital and Community Psychiatry* 32 (1981): 497-498.

4. M. L. Lanza, "The Reactions of Nursing Staff to Physical Assault by a Patient," *Hospital and Community Psychiatry* 34 (1983): 44-47.

5. G. Pisarcik, "Why Patients Use the Emergency Department," *Journal of Emergency Nursing* 6 (1980): 16-21.

6. B. D. Sales, T. D. Overcast, and K. J. Merrikin, "Worker's Compensation Protection for Assault and Batteries on Mental Health Professionals," in *Assaults Within Psychiatric Facilities*, eds. J. Lion and W. Reid (New York: Grune and Stratton, 1983).

7. J. L. Krupnick, "Victims of Violence: Psychological Responses, Treatment Implications," *Evaluation and Change,* Special Issue (1980): 42-47

8. J. R. Lion and S. A. Pasternak, "Countertransference Reactions to Violent Patients," *American Journal of Psychiatry* 130 (1973): 207-210.

9. A. W. Burgess and L. L. Holmstrom, *Rape: Victims of Crisis* (Bowie, Md: Robert J. Brady Co., 1974).

10. D. C. Aguilera and J. W. Messick, *Crisis Intervention: Theory and Methodology* (St. Louis, Mo: The C. V. Mosby Co., 1978).

11. L. I. Sank, "Commmunity Disasters," *American Psychologist* 334 (1979): 334-338.

12. A. Lazarus, *The Practice of Multimodal Therapy* (New York: McGraw-Hill, 1980).

13. B. Bursten et al., "Reducing Stress in a Traumatized Hospital," in *Management and Understanding of Hostage Incidents in Healthcare,*" ed. J. Turner (Memphis: Lifestyle Management Associates, Inc., 1984).

Index

A

Abduction. *See* Kidnapping

Addad, M., 34

Administration, security management, 209-223

Administrators, liability of, 6

Adolescents. *See* Childhood aggression; Violence, child/adolescent patient

Affectionate-rejecting parenting, 90

Aggression, models of, 58-63
  energy and aggression, 59
  environmental factors in, 60
  frustration and aggression, 60
  imitation of violence, 59
  instinctive aggression, 59
  territoriality of aggression, 60
  See also Childhood agression

Aggression management, nursing staff training, 213-249

Aggressive patient, drug/alcohol abuse and, 139

Aggrieved hostage-takers, 178

Alarm systems. *See* Duress systems

Albee, G.W., 35

Alcohol
  combined with drugs, 135-136
  emergency room violence and, 61

Alcohol abuse
  elderly patient, 112
  pathological intoxication, 131
  suicide and, 130
  violent behavior and, 130-131
  See also Drug/alcohol patient

Alcohol idiosyncratic intoxication, 131

Alcohol withdrawal delirium, 131

Allen, N., 19-20, 28

Alvarado, R., 158, 162

Alzheimer type of dementia, 109, 110

Amphetamines, violence and, 132-133

Anderson, K., 125

Angst, J., 135

Antipsychotic medication, emergency room patient, 70-71

Antisocial personality, as hostage-taker, 184

Anxiety disorders, childhood aggression and, 94

Armao, B.V., 126

Arraignments, bedside, 157

Auerbach, S., 180